Camering: Fernand Deligny on Cinema and the Image

Media / Art / Politics

The **series in Media / Art / Politics** stimulates cutting-edge research in the fields of media, arts and politics, focusing on transformations in technology, cultural expressions and political processes, and their intertwinement, in our everyday, increasingly media-saturated and globalised world. We welcome publications that address the myriad ways in which media-technological developments frame, shape and transform our (current) socio-cultural and political order, and give rise to new political ecologies, identities and communities, as well as to novel forms of cultural expression and communication. We seek to publish research that is case-based and theory-driven. However diverse the cases addressed, the studies in this series converge, in that they all take a specific set of cultural phenomena as a focal point to broach the larger socio-cultural and political issues from the perspective of a critical (media) theory in development. Art probes the implications of such changes, offering an excellent starting point for critical reflections that seek to untangle the pivotal role of media in our world today.

Other titles in this series

Inge van de Ven, Big Books in Times of Big Data, 2019

Ali Shobeiri, Place; Towards a Geophilosophy of Photography, 2021

Camering: Fernand Deligny on Cinema and the Image

Introduced and edited by Marlon Miguel
Translated by Sarah Moses
Postface by Elena Vogman

LEIDEN UNIVERSITY PRESS

The publication of this volume was made possible by

EUR ArTeC (Cet ouvrage a beneficie d'une aide de l'ANR au titre du programme Investissement d'avenir (ANR-17-EURE-0008))

Centre National du Livre (CNL)

Project "Madness, Media, Milieus. Reconfiguring the Humanities in Postwar Europe", Bauhaus-Universität Weimar/ VolkswagenStiftung

 The images were provided by the private archives of Gisèle Durand (the archives of Deligny's Network), as well as those of Any Durand, stored in Monoblet. Images/sequence of images from pages 34, 35, 36, 37, 54, 76, 102, 112, 164, 172, 234, and cover previously appeared in *Camérer. À Propos d'images*, edited by Sandra Alvarez de Toledo, Anaïs Masson, Marlon Miguel, Marina Vidal-Naquet, Paris, L'Arachnéen, 2021.

Media / Art / Politics, volume 3

Translation: Sarah Moses
Cover image: Le Serret living area, end of 1970s.
Cover design: Andre Klijsen
Lay-out: Friedemann Vervoort

ISBN 978 90 8728 384 1
e-ISBN 978 94 0060 430 8
NUR 652
Printed and bound by CPI Group (UK) Ltd, Croydon, CR0 4YY

Contents

What I can say, now that I'm in my eighty-third year, is that the images in the darkest depths of my being behave like swamp beasts; they kill and then devour each other, or rather, they devour each other alive, or copulate when they come across another of their kind. Hence the fact that I have never been able to accept the unconscious as Freud sees it; the space was taken. I'm moved when I find these images alive and moving inside me again—moved to tears that never flow. I have never heard the images that haunt us spoken of; they seize me when I lend myself to their proliferating presence; I'm then very far from others and ready to write. Sometimes, I get down to it, as I have just now, my hand as strange as everything I can see, and animated by convulsive movements that lead it down familiar paths; at the heart of these movements, the vivid image that flows like lava at the heart of a volcano. But when I set out on these paths, I lose whomever it is that reads me. I have to return to the universe that is customary to them, even if it means setting out towards the image once again, if the story presents me with a fissure in which to do so.[1]

1 The epigraph is excerpted from a text stored at the Institut Mémoires de l'édition contemporaine (IMEC) and was partially published in French as 'Un prof' in *Camérer. À propos d'images*, Paris, L'Arachnéen, 2021. Likely written in 1996, the text concerns Deligny's secondary school philosophy teacher, who was shot in the courtyard of the Citadel de Lille in 1942.

Translator's Note

Sarah Moses

In the epigraph to this volume, Fernand Deligny tells of being 'moved to tears that never flow' by the images alive inside him, images that haunt him and seize him when he sits down to write. This image of the pedagogue, writer, storyteller, cineaste, his hand convulsing across the page—the last I translated and the first to appear in *Camering*—moved me deeply in turn; I knew I could sharpen it no further when reading his words in my English had the same effect as they did in French.

This is what I was after. As I rendered into English the images and texts that make up *Camering*, I sought a reading experience that came as close as possible to that in French. If Deligny moved the Francophone reader in one direction and not another—to laughter rather than tears, to wonder and not indifference, to insight instead of bafflement; if his words stirred or stilled them, invited them to linger or urged them along, helped them get their bearings or get lost—my hope is that he will similarly affect the Anglophone reader.

In a volume that gathers his ideas on the image and cinema, capturing with English words what he depicts so vividly and viscerally was key to reproducing the reading experience. Deligny's images were among the most poetic passages in *Camering*, and perhaps as such my favourite to translate. When I sit down to write this note, and consider the approach I took, I see certain of them in sharp detail again. I see, for example, the Pentecost procession in the streets of Lille when Deligny was a child, which he describes in 'Miscreating':

> the parade of floats, small troupes of jolly fellows and giants, veritable monuments, and ambulant scaffolding cloaked in multicoloured fabrics atop which sat masques that were smiling and fuming, of characters legendary and familiar.

I treated passages such as this as I would poetry, looking for the rhythms and patterns of sound that give it its texture, and then seeking to reproduce them in translation. Thus the sentence, itself a parade—of images—contains many of the same sounds and stresses as the French: *troupes de joyeux drilles et des géants* became 'troupes of jolly fellows and giants' and *un masque souriant et furibard* became 'masques that were smiling and fuming'.

It was also key to reproduce Deligny's idiosyncratic style: he can be both serious and playful, formal and colloquial, conceptual and poetical; he tends towards idiom, wordplay, irony, and humour. In translating him, I was guided by a principle of sorts—not to normalise in English what in French was anything but. This meant embracing unexpected and at times unwieldy, circuitous, and fragmentary sentences to mirror Deligny's syntactical choices. Lexically, it meant opting for unfamiliar words and rare or anachronistic uses to mirror his often uncommon choices in French. It also entailed coming up with new words for neologisms such as the verb *camérer*, which gives this volume its title. Though his choice of the infinitive form here and elsewhere, such as with *mécréer*, 'miscreating', is intentional and important—precisely because the form is tenseless—in English the gerund was necessary grammatically when the French infinitive functioned as a noun. Conversely, when Deligny used the gerund as a neologism for an individual who carried out a particular activity—*camérant* is both the present participle of 'to camer' and the person who camers—this verb form did not work in English and I opted for 'cameror', and elsewhere 'writor' and 'realisor', swapping the expected 'er' ending with an 'or'.

Deligny pays close attention to the workings of the French language throughout his writings. Often, this is a means of highlighting the ways language is used—and inviting the reader to question them along with him. English is, of course, not always used in similar or parallel ways to French, and certain linguistic puzzles were among the most challenging to work out as a translator. Such was the case with Deligny's treatment of the reflexive pronoun *se*—in English, 'oneself', 'itself', 'ourselves', 'themselves', etc. He frequently places *se* in italics or uppercase letters, thereby emphasising his notion that the idea one forms of the *self* limits what one can see, such as the human, or the image as he regards it. Whereas in French *se* is often necessary, the English equivalent is often not—unless, of course, it's fundamental to the notion being put forth. In 'Fossils Have a Hard Life: Apropos of the Image', for instance, Deligny writes of striking images that stir us because they're human, 'not as a result of what's seen (by the self), for it's here that the paradox lies; the human is not seen (by the *self*)'. The passive reflexive construction, *ce qui se voit* means 'what's seen', but key here is the *se*, the *self* that in French also functions as the subject of the active construction 'what the self sees', hence my decision to render it as 'what's seen (by the self)', and *l'humain ne* se *voit pas* as 'the human is not seen (by the *self*)'.

Deligny's interest in language is also evident in the ways he considers and plays with the etymology of words in his writing. He begins the first 'Camering' text in this volume with an examination of the verb *projeter*:

> Words have a history. What the dictionary told us—in times past—of *projeter*, to project, was '*jeter dehors*', the image evoked being that of rejecting something, throwing it out, while the word *projet*, a project, which has the same origin, evokes 'all that by which people tend to modify the world or themselves in a given way'.

When the roots of words were crucial to the ideas Deligny developed in a text, I included the French in italics followed or preceded by the English translation. This way, I figured, the curious reader could get a better sense of what Deligny was up to. But I also wanted the reading experience to be as fluid as possible—that is, when it was in the original. As such, I chose not to place French words, expressions, and even fragments of sentences in brackets, which I felt would have been disruptive, but instead to weave them into the English translation.

I took a similar approach to translating wordplay, in particular when it hinged on the use of sound. In 'The Alga and the Fungus', for example, Deligny plays with the homophones *la mère* and *la mer*, words that sound the same in French, but not in English, and have different meanings:

> *La mère d'Arthur Rimbaud,* the poet's mother, was quite devout; as for *la mer*, the sea, Rimbaud had never seen it when he wrote the chef-d'oeuvre on which it's based; yet when it came to *sa mère*, his mother, he was unable to see her.

On other occasions, when sound was important but not vital, I sought a translation skewed slightly in favour of it over sense, such as in 'Miscreating', where Deligny writes: *Il y avait méprise, sinon mépris. Méprise* and *mépris* are paronyms—words that are pronounced and spelt similarly but have different meanings. I translated them as 'misconception' and 'contempt', respectively, preferring this interpretation of *méprise* to the more common 'mistake' or 'misunderstanding' for the effect, however small, of the repetition of sounds between it and 'contempt'.

Wordplay that hinges on sense rather than sound also abounds in *Camering*, and polysemy was particularly tricky to replicate. Instead of choosing one meaning when there was an intentional befuddling of senses, I tried to reproduce ambiguity if at all possible. Sometimes this was easy enough to do. In 'Fossils Have a Hard Life: Apropos of the Image', for example, Deligny plays with the multiple meanings of the noun *un organe*, 'an organ'. In French, as in English, the word can signify both an instrument and a body part that carries out a function, and the ambiguity is key to Deligny's thinking. In the same text, he uses the word *métier* in a similar fashion. In this case a simple swap—'métier' for *métier*—was not an option, as in addition to the sense Anglophone readers are likely familiar with, the French word refers to a weaving loom. Here I used the italicised French word with a footnote when the original was ambiguous, and specified one or the other of the English words when it was not. Trickier still was Deligny's use of a single verb with several meanings, which varied according to context and form, rarely in the same ways as in English. As with passages where a word's etymology was important, here I interwove Deligny's French in italics with my English.

If I could not reproduce ambiguity, I asked myself if there was a way to retain multiple meanings in English. One approach I took was to translate a single word as multiple words. For example, *une dérive*, taken again from 'Fossils Have a Hard Life: Apropos of the Image' can be both 'a downward turn' and 'a drift'. Deligny also uses the word to signify a figurative movement away from the path usually followed. Rather than favouring any one of these senses, I attempted to hint at all of them with the translation 'downward drift'. The last sense is part of Deligny's lexicon—what he refers to earlier in the text as the jargon used in the métier of living close to autistic children. He considered this living experience an attempt, and it entailed 'a drift' from the well-worn path taken by institutions that at the time sought to 'heal' these children. Another of Deligny's meanings for *une derive* is of particular interest here: he used it to describe his approach to writing, which involved seeking words and language that 'drifted' from usual usages and senses.

An important word in Deligny's lexicon and in *Camering*—one with several meanings—is *un bonhomme.* The French noun often refers to 'an average bloke' or 'a good fellow', but it also denotes, among other things, 'a stickman'. Deligny makes use of these meanings, but for him *le bonhomme,* often translated here as 'the everyman', also signifies an important concept: that of the average bloke who has incorporated a generic image of what man looks like and as a consequence, cannot see. Elsewhere in *Camering*, I chose to include the French word and pair it with one of its English meanings, though readers would benefit from keeping in mind the fact that it has several. The recurrence of *un bonhomme* is significant and it would have been lost if the French had not been retained in the translation.

Throughout *Camering*, readers will come across films that are realised rather than made. Though *réaliser un film* is usually translated as 'to make a film', I chose the cognate verb for several reasons. Most important of these is the distinction Deligny makes between filming and camering. While he views the former as being driven by intentions and an end product, camering is non-subjective, endless, about the tool and the process; in short, not about making a film-object. Furthermore, 'realise' seemed the better choice because of Deligny's interest in etymology and his preference for uncommon uses of words.

Though it was my aim to enable the Anglophone reader to experience as many of the layers of Deligny's texts as were present in French, sometimes I was at a loss when it came to working them seamlessly into the translation. On these occasions, I turned to footnotes. They are intended to explain certain translation choices as well as provide biographical, historical, and linguistic context. I also included references to films and individuals Deligny discusses, and, where possible, to English translations of the works he cites.

I would like to thank Aïcha Daher, Vincent Fleifel, Luciana Ogando, and Rob Scarborough for their help clarifying the different layers of Deligny's French, and the volume's editor, Marlon Miguel, for patiently untangling the knottier sentences with me, elucidating certain of the more challenging concepts, and for the care with which he revised each of the texts that make up *Camering*.

General Introduction

Marlon Miguel

Cinema on the Margins and in the Centre of Deligny's Experiments

Cinema occupies an ambiguous position in the work of Fernand Deligny: it is both central and marginal. For Deligny, cinema constitutes a space of practice as well as one of conceptual speculation. Present to a greater or lesser degree in different periods of his life, it is nonetheless a common thread that runs through more than fifty years of clinical, pedagogical, and socio-political experimentation.

If Deligny's work has for decades been associated with pedagogy and the so-called social 'maladjustment' of children and adolescents; if as a result of the renewed interest in his work from the late 2000s[1] his writing has come to be associated with a style both conceptual and poetical, the crucial relationship it maintained with cinema and the image continues to be a blind spot. In the French clinical and cinematographic context, there has been renewed interest in certain of 'his' films, including *Le Moindre geste* (*The Slightest Gesture*, 1971) and *Ce Gamin, là* (*That Kid, There*, 1975). Yet very little has been written about the ways in which the cinematographic practice was essentially interwoven in Deligny's experiments or how speculative reflection on the image constituted a vital line of his thought.

This blind spot in the reception of Deligny's work is due first to the fact that the majority of his texts on cinema and the image have remained unpublished until now. Many were discovered only recently during the organisation of his archives.[2] *Camering: Fernand Deligny on Cinema and the Image* is a first step towards filling this gap. Its title is taken from a series of texts and notes that date from the late 1970s, which Deligny called *camérer*. Three of them, the most important and polished pieces, are published in *Camering*.

This volume reunites, in chronological order, pieces written in different styles between 1934 and 1996. They offer an overview of Deligny's involvement with cinema, beginning with a short review he wrote about three films screened at a cine-club for the journal *Lille Université*. There is a large gap between this piece and the two that follow: 'The Camera, a Pedagogical Tool' concerns Deligny's first practical experiment with the camera, while 'He's Still One of Us' is a reflection on *The Slightest Gesture*. The latter, along with the remaining texts in this volume, was written during

Deligny's most productive period, when he lived with autistic children. The reader will note that the texts become progressively more speculative and shift from work with the camera and reflections on cinema towards an unstable and mysterious notion of the 'image'. 'Miscreating', 'The Alga and the Fungus', 'Fossils Have a Hard Life: Apropos of the Image', and 'The Distinctiveness of the IMAGEs' had until recently been lost along with numerous other texts inside long-forgotten boxes, trunks, and suitcases in the attic of an old house in the Cévennes.

Deligny produced many texts on cinema and the image, among them a variety of scripts, most unpublished and now stored at the Institut Mémoires de l'édition contemporaine / The Institute for Contemporary Publishing Archives (IMEC) (see *infra*, note 75). However, the aim of this volume, far from being exhaustive, is to provide a compact and insightful glimpse into his reflections and practices in these areas. Furthermore, because of his obsessive manner of writing, many texts from the Cévennes period are similar to or intersect with one another—passages and themes reappear in different works. For this reason, the decision was made to include a selection of the most representative texts from each period, as this would enable the reader to follow the movement of and displacements in Deligny's reflection.

The gap in the reception of Deligny's work on cinema and the image can be explained by several factors. First among these is that although cameras played a central role in many of his experimental 'attempts'—*tentatives*, as he refers to them in French[3]—with delinquents and psychotic and autistic children, it was never Deligny's intention to devote himself to cinema or become a filmmaker. In fact, he generated contexts in which cinema could be practised without touching a camera himself, just as he proposed the well-known cartographic practice that entailed tracing the movements and gestures of autistic children without tracing the maps himself. In this sense, Deligny is neither a director nor a scriptwriter, and much less a historian or theoretician of cinema; his written production cannot, strictly speaking, be considered a theory of the image. Nevertheless, there is no doubt that cinema and the image can be regarded as one of the main lines with which we can approach his writings.

It is for this reason that cinema plays both a central and marginal role in Deligny's practice and his speculative reflection. He moves alongside and away from cinema; his experimentation takes form through and within cinema; he elaborates on the image to reflect on autistic perception and memory or to develop his critiques of classical humanism and discursive language, without succumbing to the temptation of post-humanist trends, and always insisting on the importance of the 'human' (species). And since the practice of cinema is invited into his different attempts, and occupies a central position in them without being vital to their survival, there is always a wide opening for experimentation. In these attempts, the energy mobilised through the cinematographic practice does not saturate the effort of creating a film-object, but is instead invested in the processes around it—processes that are always intimately connected to the other activities in the attempt, such as hosting delinquent adolescents and inventing pedagogical situations involving them, or living with autistic children and making bread or cheese together. This approach does not imply that the film itself was unimportant, but it did play a role in emancipating the work created from the temporality of traditional and commercial cinematographic production. Released from the necessity of a film-product, Deligny and the group involved in its creation could carry out the other activities inside which the project of the *film to come* would take place. At the same time, the film projects were not in any way secondary or superfluous. Nor were they conceived simply as a means of documenting these activities. On the contrary, they helped to otherwise structure Deligny's pedagogical and clinical attempts. And they played a symmetrical role by also helping to emancipate these same attempts from their supposed aim—that of healing or normalising psychotic persons, and re-educating or readjusting deviant subjects.

Deligny's Trajectory: a Life of Attempts

Deligny is a challenging figure to classify. Primarily known as an educator or pedagogue, the author himself refused the category in as early as 1967.[4] Nor is he a psychologist or a philosopher, even if he does dialogue with both fields. Later, engaging with the field of social work, he stated he would prefer to identify himself as a 'poet and ethologist'.[5] As we will see in detail, his perspective on clinical and re-educational practices is indeed closer to anthropology or even ethology. Certainly, something that characterises each of his different attempts is the fact that they were always accompanied by the practice of writing—writing that was very much the form he used to develop his experiences. Deligny is not a professional with a graduate degree, and was very sceptical of 'specialists' of all sorts, preferring always to carry out his attempts with workers, farmers, artists, 'common' people. In fact, very early on, he abandoned the bachelor's degree in philosophy and psychology he had begun in Lille, in northern France. If we follow his own narrative, instead of going to university or writing exams he preferred to 'go to the cinema'.[6]

After leaving university once and for all, Deligny soon began working in a class of children with special needs—thanks to help from the father of his friend François Châtelet, the future well-known historian of philosophy. It was the beginning of a long trajectory of work with 'abnormal' children that would continue until his very last days.

Deligny's trajectory can be broadly organised into three significant periods: 1938–1948, 1948–1962, and 1967–1996. They describe his movement from work of a more intra-institutional nature towards that which took place outside the institution.

During the first period, Deligny worked inside the main public institutions for 'maladjusted' children and adolescents: in two special classes; in a psychiatric asylum in the city of Armentières, close to Lille; and as the director of an observation centre for young delinquents in Lille. Deligny was also recruited to the armed forces for a short period between 1939 and 1940, an experience that recurs frequently in his writings.[7] This extremely ambiguous time in France, from the Front Populaire era, moving through the Vichy occupation, and arriving at liberation, was characterised by the structuring of a series of institutions, technologies, professions, and laws concerning young 'abnormal' people. The general concept of a 'maladjusted childhood',[8] established in 1943, marked the beginning of an important discontinuity in the legal, social, educational, and psychiatric fields. In a sense, it indicated the end of an era of total exclusion and confinement, and the beginning of a new one that was violent in different ways, and was based on forced inclusion.[9]

Though intra-institutional, Deligny's different attempts were aimed at disrupting the 'instituted' functions of such spaces, as well as the related operations that led to the establishment of traditional divisions, such as that between a 'normal' class and a 'special' class, the teacher who has the knowledge and the students who passively receive it—students who are themselves divided into good and bad, 'normal' and 'abnormal'—and between the warders and 'the insane'. Deligny's efforts were directed towards creating collective situations where such divisions, which were responsible for establishing the positions and thus the identities of each subject in the space, could be neutralised. Maladjusted children in a special class would become 'experts in modes of being' during storytelling sessions;[10] warders and the mentally ill were brought together for weaving sessions inside the asylum; delinquents acted in films and were involved in shooting them.

Particularly interesting is Deligny's work at the Armentières asylum. He forbid disciplinary sanctions, invited the warders and their wives to participate in activities with the patients, and organised ateliers, group sports, and walks outside the asylum. In this way, he tried to change the immutable time-space of the asylum by producing new and unexpected 'occasions' that might ultimately trigger the mentally ill patients into engaging in some activity. With these experiments, he aimed to create a network of persons, a 'collectivity', in which the usual instituted functions could change. To do so, he transformed the warders into educators of sorts—they were responsible for organising activities and using other skills unrelated to their positions (playing the accordion, crafting, constructing, etc.). Their wives, most of whom were workers in the textile industry, were asked to bring in materials and run sewing and embroidery ateliers, but also to help organise other activities, such as the reconstruction of asylum spaces. By not taking the patients as 'irrecoverable mad people', but as persons needing 'occasions' to do something, by creating a 'network' between them and the warders and their wives, and by initiating communication between the 'inside' and the 'outside', Deligny aimed at a neutralisation of the usual functioning of the asylum.[11]

Deligny further developed some of the principles he had implemented in Armentières shortly after the war, when he began to work as the director of the first Centre d'observation et de triage (literally Observation and Triage Centre), located in Lille. Created in 1945, these centres were established to observe and evaluate young delinquents for a certain period of time before the justice system could take a 'technical' decision regarding their futures—send them to prison, special schools, other re-educational organisations, etc. Deligny writes of his experiences at the centre in the 1947 book *Les Vagabonds efficaces* (*The Efficient Vagabonds*).[12] During his time there, he once again chose not to work with professional educators, but instead with individuals from working-class backgrounds. Furthermore, he transformed the centre into an open space where family members of the adolescents could visit, as could poets, musicians, and anarchists, especially during the events organised in the evenings. In his book, Deligny attacks the perspective of education conceived as a moralisation process and considers it through the lens of emancipation. He believed it was preferable to work not with highly qualified professionals, but rather with persons coming from the same social milieu as that of the young delinquents. His conception can be synthesised with a simple idea: a social milieu alone is apt to take care of itself, to think about itself, and to find the appropriate solutions to its own problems. That is why it seemed crucial to him to think in terms of creating an internal and popular network that was immanent in the social and political situation, rather than waiting for external solutions from technical professionals with their presumed know-how. What at the time was called 'educational readjustment' ought to be linked, in Deligny's perspective, to a comprehension of the social and political circumstances at stake and to the necessity of actively participating in them.

Deligny's radical position at the centre in Lille led to it being shut down less than one year after opening. He then worked for a short time at the popular educational and cultural organisation Travail et Culture (Work and Culture), alongside figures such as cinema critic André Bazin and future filmmaker Chris Marker.[13] Deligny has said of this time that it involved, among other things, 'escorting' films programmed by Travail et Culture.[14]

The following years, from 1948 to 1962, mark the second important period in Deligny's trajectory. With his then wife and communist activist Huguette Dumoulin, the support of the French Communist Party (PCF), Henri Wallon's laboratory for childhood psychobiology, and the anarchist youth hostel network—as well as, in its first years, the social security system—he created the para-institutional network of social re-education for juvenile delinquents called La Grande Cordée. The network sought 'occasions' that would give juvenile offenders something to do with their lives, and would help emancipate them from the infernal institutional cycle of maladjustment; furthermore, it sought to constitute a 'collectivity' or 'supportive milieu'[15] that they could be part of. The 'occasions' took place away from the adolescents' homes and were conceived as collective situations that would entail, for example, learning a job they took pleasure in, or developing a project. The aim was to constitute new 'conditions of existence assumed to be favourable to their development'.[16] In each case, the adolescent was sent somewhere in France for a temporary 'trial placement'.[17] If they enjoyed their time there they could stay on as an employee; otherwise, they were sent to another placement.

La Grande Cordée's conception was heavily influenced by the ideas of Soviet pedagogue Anton Makarenko, as well as by principles from the tradition of popular education—such as those developed by Célestin Freinet or by the CEMÉA (Centres d'entrainement aux méthodes d'éducation active / Training Centres in Methods of Active Education). On the one hand, Deligny was undeniably close to the Soviet and Marxist traditions—and the PCF wanted to transform him into a sort of 'French Makarenko'; on the other, he took some distance from them, particularly in emphasising that France was a post-war capitalist society, one very different from the Soviet post-revolutionary context in which Makarenko developed his experimental pedagogy at the Gorki Colony.[18] Deligny remained close to the PCF, but his libertarian position was met with some suspicion and there were those who considered him to be a 'very insufficient communist'.[19] La Grande Cordée was based in Paris and sponsored by Social Security until the beginning of the 1950s. Its structure remained more or less organised until that time. However, when the network lost its financial support in 1953, it became an itinerant group in France, and the re-education work at its core came to be increasingly mixed with the very activities that ensured its survival, such as the restoration of houses, goat farming, etc. More importantly, it was at this time that the group began to work with a camera to shoot films. The second text in this volume, 'The Camera, a Pedagogical Tool', is a crucial document of their attempt.

When La Grande Cordée dissolved, Deligny, Josée Manenti, and the last of those remaining from the group started the film project *The Slightest Gesture* (1962–1965), before Deligny was invited to La Borde clinic by Jean Oury and Félix Guattari. He spent approximately two years (1965–1967) at the clinic, largely avoiding its activities, though he was responsible for a few ateliers and cine-club sessions, and edited the journal *Cahiers de la Fgéri* (Fédération des groupes d'études et de recherches institutionnelles / Federation of Study Groups and Institutional Research). It was also at the end of 1966 that he met the autistic boy Jean-Marie J.—whom he called 'Janmari'—and that the idea for a new project involving mute autistic children began to take form.

In 1967, tired of the atmosphere at La Borde and the emphasis the clinic placed on language and verbal communication,[20] Deligny and a small group of individuals (Gisèle and Any Durand, Jacques Lin, Guy and Marie-Rose Aubert), along with Janmari, first moved to Gourgas, a property owned by Guattari in the Cévennes in southern France, and then, in 1968, to another house not far from there in the hamlet of Graniers. This was the beginning of the network of living areas conceived to host mute and severely autistic children. Though the network operated entirely outside the institution, surviving on what it produced, Deligny's books, the occasional help from local farmers, contributions from some of the children's parents, and eventually aid from a few projects and donations—in particular one made by the rock group Pink Floyd in 1973—it remained very much connected to the intellectual, cultural, and institutional landscape in France. In fact, it was Deligny's decision not to receive public support, so that there would be a larger margin for experimentation. Still, the network maintained its connections, in particular to the psychoanalytical field (and to important names such as Françoise Dolto and Maud Manonni), hosting numerous children from all over the country who had been sent by clinics or analysts. The network existed as such until 1986 and Deligny, along with Jacques Lin and Gisèle Durand, continued to work with autistic individuals until his last days in 1996.

During this period, Deligny's language underwent a radical transformation and his production increased exponentially. The majority of the texts included in this volume were written in the Cévennes. Deligny constantly plays with language, moves between biography, fiction, poetic description, and conceptual and highly speculative reflection, searches for unusual and long-forgotten words, creates numerous neologisms, and invents a strange syntax. And, indeed, his thought—but also his biography, which he ceaselessly takes over and rewrites throughout his texts and over the years—is indissociable from the language he invented in an attempt to translate the radical experience of living with children outside the reign of speech. This language is certainly all his own, but it plays within his native tongue, French, exposing its mechanisms, vices, modes of functioning, and structures, and is in dialogue with its literary tradition, with authors that implicitly or explicitly inhabit his texts, such as Stéphane Mallarmé, Arthur Rimbaud, and Francis Ponge.

Beyond what Deligny narrates and how he constantly fictionalises his own biography, his experiments are to be read as part of certain pedagogical and clinical 'utopias' that emerged and were developed in the twentieth century, in particular in the post-war period. Though Deligny's is a singular position within this horizon, one that merits further analysis, his experiments cannot be read outside the particular space between Lacanian psychoanalysis,[21] the anti-psychiatry movement, *désaliénisme* (deinstitutionalisation and 'sectorisaton'), institutional psychotherapy, and the idea of the *collectif soignant* (healing collective); between popular, radical, and emancipatory education projects. And it is mainly within these two fields—clinical and educational—that he operated in a direct manner, in particular because of the public with whom he worked. This does not mean, however, that his writings can be reduced to these fields alone; on the contrary, they take inspiration from diverse disciplines (including anthropology, the arts, philosophy, and politics) and contribute to the debates in these fields, as is evidenced by the remarkable number of interlocutors he had throughout his life: François Truffaut, Chris Marker, and Robert Kramer; Louis Althusser, Gilles

Deleuze, Marcel Gauchet, and Isaac Joseph; Maud Mannoni and Françoise Dolto, to name just a few.[22] This interdisciplinary arc can be explained, on the one hand, by his work's concern with the very status of the 'human'—a keyword in his thought—and, on the other, by his invention of a language capable of critically rethinking the conception of the human: How are normality and abnormality defined? How does one trace where the human begins and ends? And by allying himself with 'the mad, the delinquents, the retarded, the dissidents',[23] by de-solidarising himself with that which was 'similar'[24]—his *semblables*, other human beings in general—and with the dominant 'image of Man',[25] Deligny developed, as we will see in his writings, a radical anthropological and political critique of resemblance, similitude, likeness.

The fact that Deligny's name was largely forgotten in the final decades of the last century can perhaps be linked to the coincident end of clinical and educational utopias such as those mentioned above. However, the rediscovery of his work that has begun to take place in recent years demonstrates the current relevance of his thought and is an opportunity to better grasp it today.

The Camera as a Tool

The practice of cinema, or what could, strictly speaking, be regarded as the use of the camera, first became part of Deligny's attempts during the period of La Grande Cordée. The archives from these years show that cameras were included in the budgets of Deligny's first funding applications for the network. In as early as 1950, he was able to acquire a 16 mm Paillard camera, but he likely only began shooting with the adolescents in the group in 1952. A screening of some of the images they had captured was organised in Paris in 1954, and other sequences were shot in 1955 and 1956. 'The Camera, a Pedagogical Tool' was written in the summer of 1955 and constitutes a sort of manifesto, while reflecting on the group's on-going film projects. Though none of these projects would be concluded, they remained central to La Grande Cordée and many ideas developed at this time were carried over to the making of *The Slightest Gesture*.

Even at this stage, Deligny emphasised the tool, a notion he would develop further with the neologism 'camering'. He did not conceive of the camera as an instrument for documentation, but as a tool that one wields and that mediates collective relationships. He saw it as not only 'for recording pedagogical activity, but for participating in this activity, a little like a lone, unique, and valued mechanical weapon in combat'.[26] Deligny's conception of La Grande Cordée was clear: rather than 'assist' the adolescents, he sought to support them and 'intervene'[27] in a way that would allow them to articulate a language and formulate their intentions and problems; in sum, to express themselves: 'Each one of them is, as much as possible, scriptwriter, stage director, author of the shots. The film is first and foremost the work of those whose lives are filmed.'[28] In an unpublished letter to Truffaut, who had planned to take part in the subsequent film project that began in 1958, and from then on was entitled *La vraie vie* (*The Real Life*), Deligny was once again explicit about his position: 'the film I plan is not a work inspired by or gleaned from the four or ten lads living here [...] The presence of the camera among lads like those I recruit seems necessary to materialise [*concrétiser*] a way of thinking, of situating oneself.'[29]

Deligny's position was thus that the film should consist in *their* work. The radicality of his gesture is twofold. First, though cinema became a central preoccupation of popular education movements after the end of the war, the focus remained primarily on educating the spectator's gaze.[30] Deligny, on the contrary, insisted on the practice, on the importance of handling the camera oneself. Second, it was not just a question of a production by non-professionals—something that in itself was rare during that period—but of one led by 'abnormal', 'marginal', 'maladjusted' adolescents. The production, Deligny felt, should be a means of exposing the origins of these adolescents, their histories and difficulties; in sum, a means for them to finally occupy a position of visibility in a society that has always rejected them. In a sense, Deligny anticipated problems that a decade later would become central to collectives such as the Medvedkin Group.[31]

Most of the adolescents hosted by La Grande Cordée had critical language learning deficits. Deligny believed producing images to be a strategy that could help them with expression. But he felt the camera could play an even deeper role by helping them to perceive reality differently, to better understand their own intentions. 'The camera wielded by the adolescents themselves helps them to see.'[32] Indeed, behind the idea of the 'supportive milieu' that defined La Grande Cordée, one sees that of the 'existence dispositive' capable of transforming the adolescents—transforming their perceptions and awareness, as well as their positions, so that they could move from the passive objects of clinical, legal, and social knowledge towards active subjects who produced knowledge, told themselves their own histories.

The word 'dispositive' is recurrent in the texts and notes from this period.[33] It resonates with Michel Foucault's use of the word many years later; i.e., it is conceived through its 'strategic nature', in response to 'an *urgent need*', 'assuming that it is a matter of a certain manipulation of relations of forces, either developing them in a particular direction, blocking them, stabilising them, utilising them'.[34]

In Deligny's case, the dispositive is regarded as a means of transforming the adolescents by 'putting order to their intentions, re-establishing a balance perturbed by the absence of concrete projects'.[35] In other words, the dispositive aims at a double transformation: first, as already indicated, to help the adolescents, in their confusion, find their 'true' intentions, and thus enable them to focus their energies into a concrete project; second, to help them understand that their problems, which are linked to the label of 'maladjustment', can only be tackled collectively, since they are intimately related to a political conjuncture that is much more structural in the context of a country where nothing but the adolescents' 'exploitation as unstable labourers is conscientiously planned'.[36] As we will see, the word 'dispositive' also plays a role in how the camera was used in the network for autistic children.

Deligny took a materialist stance—he was reading Makarenko during this period, but also Lenin (*Materialism and Empirio-criticism*), and his interlocutors were members of the Communist Party—and the dispositive aimed at a transformation that was indissociable from the development of a sort of class consciousness, self-reflection, and growing awareness. But a process of transformation such as that which Deligny sought with the dispositive needed to be anchored in a collective practice: the film.

'The Camera, a Pedagogical Tool' gives hints of at least three different film projects: (1) in the Vercors region, fifteen adolescents, along with two survivors of the Resistance, shoot traces of the Maquis from the Second World War; (2) the adolescents shoot what they see from their original social milieu and consider how their perception has changed after spending some time 'elsewhere', in a new 'living regime'; (3) they put together different sequences in order to form something that could constitute a 'unified memory' of La Grande Cordée collectivity. Other projects would be developed in the following years, but none would be completed. These projects were conceived to be more or less self-managed, with the adolescents alternating between the different aspects of film production and technical apprenticeship (handling the camera, loading film, cutting, scriptwriting, acting, etc.). They learnt these aspects of filmmaking progressively and in cooperation, the most experienced adolescents generally teaching the new ones. The pedagogical potential of the camera was thus in allowing individuals to work together to resolve tensions and problems that appeared during the production and realisation of the film.

It is again interesting to note the particular stance Deligny took. Like many of his contemporaries, he acknowledged both the 'omnipresence of modern techniques of dissemination'[37] and the 'latent danger' of images. This danger was related to the fact that 'film gives an initial impression of reality directly reproduced—a reality extracted from natural reality'.[38] But Deligny differed from his contemporaries in that he imagined a sort of *cine-pharmakon*. His position, echoing Marxist theses, was that individuals who learn to master the technique and understand how the filmic object is produced will be in a better position to resist alienation. Deligny viewed, at least during this period, cinema as a language, with its rules and usages, and said of the adolescents in La Grande Cordée: 'They can only truly know this if they try the "language" out themselves in order to perceive it without becoming spellbound by it'.[39] In this sense, cinema represented for Deligny both the danger of alienation as the result of the magical power of images and the solution if it was practised.[40]

Deligny held that the film as a *work in common* could synthesise the materialisation of the individual project with the memory of the collectivity, reunifying a group that was dispersed in several trial placements and that for this reason did not 'lend itself well to the establishment of customs and traditions that, via attitudes, transmit the collective experience from individual to individual'.[41] He felt the film should produce this aimed-at unity through the scattered stories and lived experiences of the group members; that it should become, if we take Vertov's words, a sort of 'montage of life itself'.[42]

This montage of life, this memory of the collectivity, was conceived as an indefinite, on-going process—or rather, as a 'permanent one'. Indeed, Deligny's project appears inside an interesting dialectics of two statements: the *film to come* (or, following his own expression, the *film à faire*,[43] 'to be made') and 'permanent cinema'.[44] These two statements inscribe Deligny's political project in a very experimental and speculative field. The project is thus a question of a permanent film to come, one that elaborates itself and evolves from day to day, according to its own precarity; in a sense, we could regard it as 'imperfect cinema'.[45] Such ideas emphasise the process of making and, once again, the materiality of the tool—the camera, even when used 'without film',[46] structures and sets up pedagogical action and installs the milieu *there*, where it is wielded. The camera is primarily responsible for establishing a new form of mediation between the members of the group and installing a scene and milieu.[47]

Minor Gestures

'The Camera, a Pedagogical Tool' ends with the critique of a language whose 'small and big words' are too embedded in the 'hypocrisy of bourgeoisie morale'. At the end of 1957, Deligny would meet Yves Guignard, a 'severely retarded' adolescent with psychotic traits. Yves's parents had entrusted him to Deligny's care and their encounter marked the beginning of an important turning point in Deligny's reflection, practice, and writing, one that would only be fully realised when, several years later, he met Janmari and they moved to the Cévennes. Both language and image would start to become central nodal points in his speculative work.

As already indicated, none of the film projects that Deligny began during the period of La Grande Cordée were finished. More than a decade would pass before the first cinematographic work, *The Slightest Gesture*, would be completed. The film we know today is the result of a long process. The first stage entailed shooting, which largely took place between 1962 and 1965 in the Cévennes region, though other scenes were shot at La Borde clinic. During this time, Deligny also made some attempts at cutting the film. Josée Manenti was responsible for wielding the 16 mm Paillard camera and shooting the images; Guy Aubert—an orphan who had been integrated into the Grande Cordée group years before—recorded the heart of the film's 'musical material', i.e., Yves's delirious speeches, in the evenings;[48] Any Durand wrote a simple script and also appeared in the movie; Deligny organised drawing and language development sessions with Yves, followed shooting from a peripheral position, and sometimes gave the adolescent suggestions about what he might do on camera. The second stage was that of montage, which took place years later, between 1968 and 1970, and was carried out by Jean-Pierre Daniel with the support and advice of Chris Marker.[49] It also involved the fundamental soundtrack work by Aimé Agnel and sound engineer Jean-Pierre Ruh, who mixed Yves's speeches with sounds from the Cévennes landscape, the stock market, and street demonstrations. The final cut generated a very powerful disjunction between sound and image, transforming the speech into an uncontrollable flow of words that traverses the film. This element was crucial for Deligny, and corresponded with his proposition of a discourse that would not belong to a single subject even though there was a subject who 'took the floor' and pronounced the words.[50]

One could of course think here of Deleuze's interpretation of Pier Paolo Pasolini's reflection on free indirect speech—or, as he puts it, the way modern cinema is characterised by 'breaking with uniformity on the interior monologue to replace it by the diversity, the deformity, the otherness of a free indirect discourse'.[51] Indeed, *The Slightest Gesture* works with this disruption by creating a discontinuity between image and speech, which it takes even further by linking the non-stop flow of human speech to different non-human sounds, by breaking the unity between the discourse and that of the interior monologue. Yves is not a 'subject of enunciation', but he emerges from within 'his' discourse. He takes over things he has heard on the radio or that were said by a neighbour, from De Gaulle's discourses to prayers. But by breaking the supposed unity of the discourse, Deligny aims at emphasising the 'speech that makes us what we are [...] and that reigns, universal, historical, demonstrative, zany, deadly'.[52] Written in the Cévennes in 1971, 'He's Still One of Us' already showed evidence of a concept that would later be central to Deligny's thought: the 'deadly', *meurtrière*, dimension of speech, especially when it exercises its totalising power of speaking (for) the other. The text was published that year and resonates with its context. For example, one could consider Jean-Pierre Faye's *Langage totalitaires* (1972), and the discursive and narrative method of analysis he proposes not of 'what men say but in order to pay attention to the figures that describe the *circulation* of words'.[53] Faye's method serves as a means to identify how the deadly words and syntactic chains that constitute fascist language are disseminated.

With *The Slightest Gesture*, what was previously a pedagogical tool first came to be perceived as a clinical tool of sorts, one that could help establish a link and mediate between Yves and Manenti–Deligny. For three years, they followed him, filming his erratic gestures, movements, and wanderings across the Cévennes landscape. They did not have many rolls of film, the shots were taken once, the 'scenes' were not repeated, and the film seemed to evolve rather spontaneously; it was constantly reinvented as a result of the spaces they were in and the relationship established between Yves and the objects, people, and situations he encountered. In this sense, the main material of the film is precisely Yves's body in contact with the things he finds in his driftings;

it is the experimentation of his singular body in space and in touch with stones, rivers, trees, construction sites and their machines, villages and their inhabitants. What appears in the film is Yves's infinitely small world and the way his gestures are triggered by different things; the quality and repetition of these gestures. There is an interpenetration between his body, his perception, and the things in the space and his psyche—a sort of commonality of things that is explored throughout the movie and presented to the viewer.

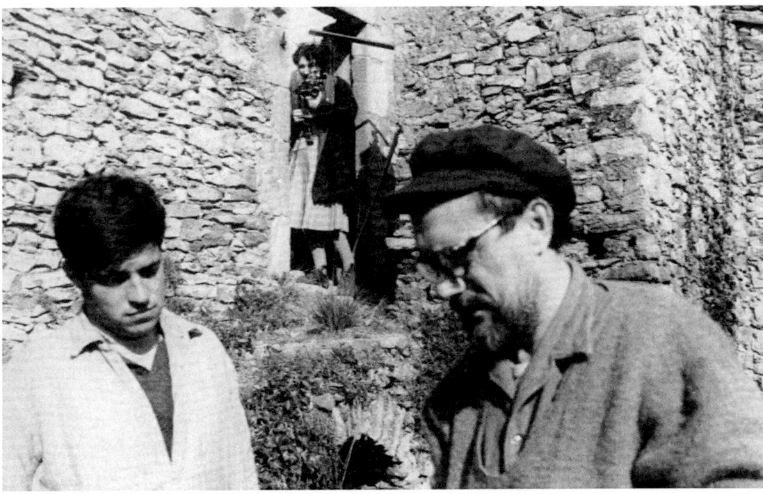

Image from the shooting of *The Slightest Gesture*.

I would claim that Daniel's approach to montage involved using certain images as 'motifs'; these would come to punctuate and give rhythm to the simple narrative. I think in particular of several images of holes in walls—which in a sense translate both the question of a 'fractured' (or 'dismantled') body and that of the autistic and 'holed' image; of houses in ruins without roofs—which one could associate with Sigmund Freud's definition of psychosis, i.e., an 'unconscious open to the sky';[54] of Yves's relentless attempts to tie his shoelaces or unknot ropes—which resonate with an idea later developed by Deligny of 'endless' gestures; of a sort of 'infinitive acting' characteristic of autistic children or of persons non-inscribed in the discourse. Of course, none of this is intentionally presented as such by Daniel, but, through montage, he found ways of expressing many of Deligny's preoccupations, which would later become central in his work with autistic children.

In his writings, Deligny frequently returned to *The Slightest Gesture*, commenting on it, and occasionally criticising Daniel's cut by calling into question whether it was radical enough, as he does, for example, in 'Miscreating', where he emphasises that more time devoted to Yves's attempts at tying knots was needed. Despite Deligny's regrets, there is no doubt that the movie remains a sort of paradigmatic object of what could be considered his cinematographic conception.

Furthermore, the movie accomplishes something that had been germinating since La Grande Cordée: it is the result of a real collective process, one which makes it very difficult to identify the author—is it Manenti? Daniel? Deligny? Yves?; a process based on a certain economy, simplicity, 'poverty' of resources. Deligny's position on this poverty is related in part to his resistance to the commercial, technological, and spectacle-based cinematographic model. But he also believes that a 'poverty' of resources constitutes the necessary means to open breaches in the director's field of intentionality, and can create a space where coincidence and unpredictability can occur. Against the representation of model-bodies, of certain normative types of affectivity and behaviour, Deligny felt that chance could constitute the principle of a practice capable of interrupting anticipation and pre-given signification. I will return to these subjects later, but for now, I want to emphasise that far from the idea of representing Yves, *The Slightest Gesture* takes a completely different track: by making it possible to perceive his gestures, attitudes, corporality, it aims at revealing his particular body, his 'way of being', his singular *mode of existence*.

The Slightest Gesture is the story of these odd gestures, which one might feel lack something, and in which the link between a certain action and the one that would 'naturally' follow is broken. From the perspective of 'normality', these gestures may appear unfinished, without reason or aim. And it is precisely to contradict this perspective, to show its limitation, that the movie focuses on these *minor* gestures.

The Other Gravity: Deligny's Anthropological Position

Deligny's late reflection on the image and cinema cannot be separated from the work carried out by the network for mute autistic children he established in the Cévennes in the summer of 1967. The Cévennes attempt was not founded on principles of a healing treatment or cure, and Deligny constantly dismisses such terms in his discourse. Certainly, it involved a clinical process of sorts, but one that was completely diluted in ordinary tasks such as taking care of the space, farming, bread production, etc. Along with these tasks, special attention was given to space and to the placement of objects in it, as well as to the precise organisation of schedules for what had to be done—what Deligny calls 'the customary'. In this sense, the various living spaces in the network were really thought of as installations where everything had its time and place. Each living area generally housed one to three adults, as well as between two and six autistic children. The network was most active during the 1970s, when for a time it consisted of seven different living areas, housed around ten children on a permanent basis, and hosted as many as thirty or forty during the summer.

For Deligny, the main problem concerning autistic individuals was the standard psychiatric approach at the time, which expected them to be, become, and behave exactly like those we consider 'normal'. That is why, through a particular rhetoric, Deligny prefers to think of autistic children not as 'abnormal' or 'handicapped', but as manifesting another 'mode of being' (*mode d'être*), belonging to another 'structure', living under 'another gravity'. Thus, he proposes we learn the conditions and circumstances in which these children can live well and exercise their own 'normativity'.[55]

Deligny refuses to follow the path of comparison—to compare autistic mute children to speaking subjects. Nor does he take that of analogy; that is, of translating the children's absence of speech into a form that could replace this 'gap' in order to make them efficient, or that constitutes some capacity analogous to this 'absence', 'privation', or 'lack' of speech.[56] For this reason, Deligny puts forth a very interesting notion of the 'human', conceptualised through its plasticity and 'diversity of forms'.[57] With it, he proposes that the mute autistic children living in the network be regarded as individuals that are a different actualisation of the 'human'. In his system of thought, the notion of the 'human' is placed in opposition to that of the 'Man-that-we-are'. The latter emphasises the fact that every attempt to define 'Man' is limited, always situated in a specific place, time, and context, and a narcissistic projection of oneself, of what one considers to be similar. It is in this projection that a process Deligny calls *semblabilisation*, 'similarisation', takes place. The neologism names the assimilation that occurs when one takes the other to be alike or similar to oneself.[58] Through 'similarisation', one tends to project one's own image onto the other, wanting the other to be like oneself. And, as he remarks, speech is indeed the primary force enabling one to proceed in this manner: speaking is a way to assimilate, to colonise, the other.[59]

That is why, according to Deligny, the most dangerous mistake one can make when dealing with autistic children is to compare them to or regard them as 'subjects'—if one understands the subject to be an individual inscribed in the discourse, structured by signifying speech. What may seem a humanistic, well-intentioned position—that of considering the other as a subject, a similar being—in fact conceals a violent form of assimilation, a forced and brutal operation of inclusion. From a practical, clinical, ethical, but also aesthetic perspective, this critical position has consequences. Deligny notes that as autistic mute children are not able to speak, they do not organise and represent the world as speaking subjects do; they do not live in a properly signifying dimension and the modes they develop to establish relations with the world thus function according to radically different forms.

In order to avoid 'similarisation', Deligny adopts the position of insisting on the transformation of oneself—the 'normal' speaking subject—rather than that of the autistic child. We can affirm, for this reason, that his position is anthropological rather than psychiatric. He claims in his 1975 book, *Nous et l'Innocent* (*Us and the Innocent*), that 'each individual is the first, a human, no more, no less than the very first humans that opened the way to this species'.[60] He thus underlines the perfectibility and the incomparability of each individual. That is why the 'attempt' is structured as a sort of perspectival principle: 'What was at stake this time was to look at language from the "position" of a mute child as it is possible to look at justice from the window of a delinquent child'.[61] Or, as he puts it in a letter to Althusser: 'What is the object of our practice? This or that psychotic child? Certainly not. The real object that is to be transformed is "us", "us, there", close to these "subjects" that strictly speaking are hardly subjects'.[62]

It is in this context, in 1969, that 'cartography' first appeared as a tool of experimentation in the network. Unsure how to deal with the children's crises, Deligny suggested that the 'close presences'—the non-professional speaking adults who resided with the autistic children in the network's various living areas—retreat from action, from direct intervention in their behaviours. Instead of actively doing something, he proposed that they back away and 'trace' the children's movements, wanderings, and gestures in space. In a sense, the maps' appearance in the network was related first to a clinical strategy to 'distract' the close presences and put them in another state of presence and 'observation'. Isaac Joseph, the sociologist and key Deligny collaborator, put it precisely when he described the maps as a tool to control the 'therapeutic anxiety' experienced by the close presences.[63]

'Map' and 'cartography' are in fact wide-ranging categories that englobe the different drawings traced by the close presences. There are maps of gestures and movements, of objects, a small room, a large territory; some describe a specific event, others series of actions. Usually they concern one child, but they can also describe several individuals in a specific space. They are often diachronic, so that we see several actions in the space, but they also frequently have a narrative. The maps are different sizes and formats and were made in function of the available material. Often a base map was first traced and then over it, on a superposed piece of carbon paper, the lines that described the movements, so that one could see the different layers of time, space, and the 'common', collective, progression. Deligny specifies the movements of the autistic children with the term *lignes d'erre*, often translated as 'wander lines', despite the fact that *erre* evokes instead the movement of a ship when it ceases to be mechanically propelled.[64] Indeed, the term *erre* reveals a good deal about both the close presences' attitude—of not directing, or guiding, the children's behaviour—and the children's movements, which were certainly characterised by a wandering quality, but made possible because they were inscribed within a specific territory; *erre* also means 'trace', a 'way of moving forward' and is a homophone of *aire* (*aire de séjour*, 'living area').[65]

If the maps first appeared as a means of disrupting the therapeutic drive, they quickly became an important tool that helped the close presences install the space—that is, position themselves in it, perceive things they would not have without these apparatuses, and constantly rearrange them. The cartographies played another role as what could be considered an art of memory, enabling the close presences to remember where each item belonged—which was important clinically in that it helped organise the space and ease the children's crises.[66] In this sense, the installed spaces worked as therapeutic machines of sorts, allowing the autistic children to organise their bodies and their perception. At the same time, they allowed the close presences to serve a certain function, one capable of mobilising the children's attention, thus helping them unify their sensorial experiences, and become better able to act.

In order to serve this function, the close presences lived in a very ritualised manner. This can clearly be observed in the films, for example in *That Kid, There*. One sees the constancy and a certain aesthetics in the close presences' gestures, the very precise rhythm imposed on daily tasks—even the simplest ones such as preparing a snack or washing the dishes—as if actions were choreographed and 'adorned'.

It is interesting to note that if the space constituted a key element in the 'clinical' process, this was also because it enabled a more indirect approach to being with the children and a suspension of the knowledge assumed about them. The close presences mediated their relationships with the children and the 'care' they provided through the space. In *That Kid, There*, one sees precisely how there was very little 'inter-subjectivity' in the ordinary sense, very little in the way of a direct relationship between those staying in the living areas. In the film's images, one often sees the close presences giving the impression of being absent or inattentive; in fact, an entirely different sort of 'attention' and listening is being developed—a type of attention akin to being 'on standby', a presence without being excessively present. The aim was to build this fragile dialectics of distance-closeness capable of both respecting the incommensurable distance of alterity and pursuing the effort of forging bonds—of accepting the distance and at the same time being closely present, creating a zone of proximity where the autistic child felt safe and was encouraged to act.[67]

Camering

It is noteworthy that the hosting of autistic children and the daily activities in the network were accompanied by the colossal production of all sorts of documentation: journals, letters, photos, drawings, maps, texts, and films (video, super 8, 16, and 35 mm). This living archive aimed not at representing the children, but at multiplying perspectives. In the case of the cartography, it is important to mention that the multiple layers of the maps were aimed at an erasure of subjective identities, even at the impossibility of determining who was who in a certain territory: Was the trace that of a speaking subject or an autistic child? And, in each case, which individual among the many living there? The layers also made it impossible to discern who traced the map and who 'performed' the actions in the territory.[68] In this sense, these different forms of documentation certainly involved an observational component, but they were not conceived of as instruments to produce a positive theory on autism or psychosis. Rather, they were meant to suspend the supposed neutral exterior of psychiatric and diagnostic knowledge on 'abnormal' individuals. They constituted 'reflexive' tools used in a very specific situation and were aimed at completely disrupting the usual forms of representation. Reflexivity and multiple archivisation are thus to be considered inside a collective practice of 'perspectivism', of the invention of a world—something that always implies a degree of fiction, though a fiction does not produce something that is 'fictive'.[69] This practice was indissociable from the aimed-at transformation of this 'us, there', as Deligny mentioned to Althusser.

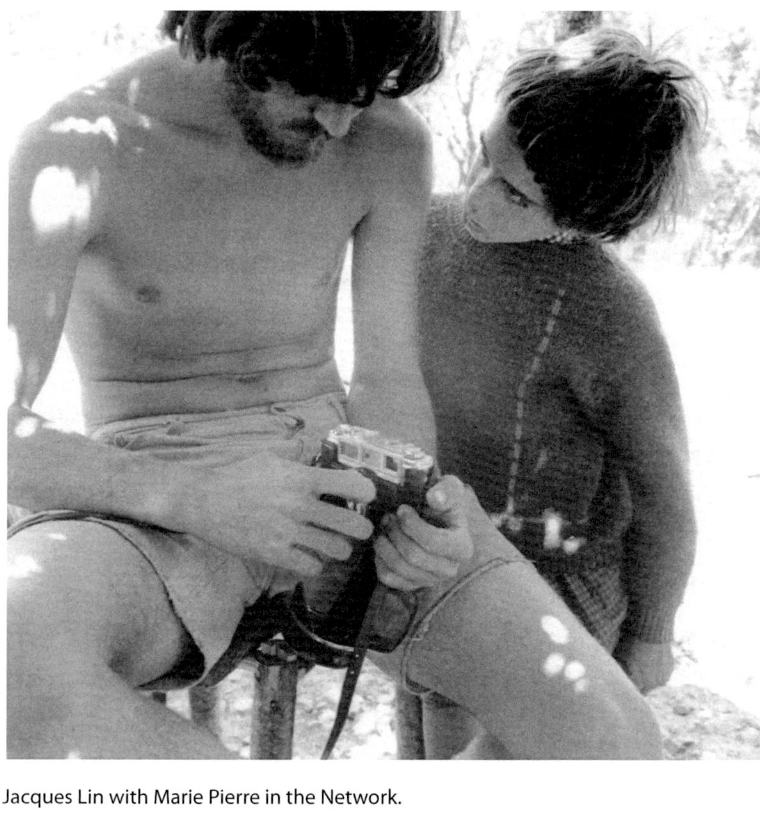

Jacques Lin with Marie Pierre in the Network.

Deligny occupied an interesting and ambiguous place in the network. On the one hand, he did not produce these different documents; he did not move between the living area he resided in (Graniers) and the others in the network; and the different close presences had the complete freedom to carry out their everyday lives and experiment in their areas as they saw fit. On the other hand, Deligny was undoubtedly the 'storyteller',[70] the person who conceptualised and proposed the different *dispositives*, and the nodal point and mediator between the living areas—which did not communicate much among themselves but directly with him—as well as between the inner world of the network and external work. This explains the very intricate and collaborative nature of what took place in the network and gave it its specificity. Deligny was completely dependent on the remarkably inventive work of the close presences and the material they produced—this is precisely what constituted the subject matter of his storytelling—while they were dependent on his ideas and proposals to keep working and inventing. Publications such as the three *Cahiers de l'Immuable* (*The Notebooks of the Immutable*) clearly evidence the complex entanglement and collaborative form of work developed there.[71] And as for Deligny's own texts, they also constitute a multiplicity of sorts: they consist of conceptual, speculative, and poetic works, letters, fictions (scripts, plays, novels, stories), biographic texts, and numerous pieces that mix these diverse genres.

At the end of the 1970s, when the cartographic practice began to fade away before it was completely abandoned in around 1980, the use of the camera—which had persisted as a tool from the start—became even more central in the network and started to occupy a dominant place in Deligny's reflections.

Cameras were regularly wielded in the network for different purposes. First, as a means of documenting the children's activities, very often in super 8 format, the result of which was destined mainly for their families. This close collaboration with the children's families was indeed an important characteristic of the network and followed a principle of 'transmission': the aim was that the majority of the children return to their original living milieus and homes, and that there, the families adapt the techniques, the 'therapeutic machines', that had been developed with each child in the network and had been proven favourable.

Second, shooting was a parallel practice to cartography, one that accompanied the daily activities, but that was not exactly destined for the children's parents. Over the years, Jacques Lin, in particular, produced a large amount of material—including frame-by-frame short animation works, such as *Les fossiles ont la vie dure* (1994), which shares its title with one of the texts included in this volume ('Fossils Have a Hard Life: Apropos of the Image'). Lin continued to shoot even after Deligny's death.[72]

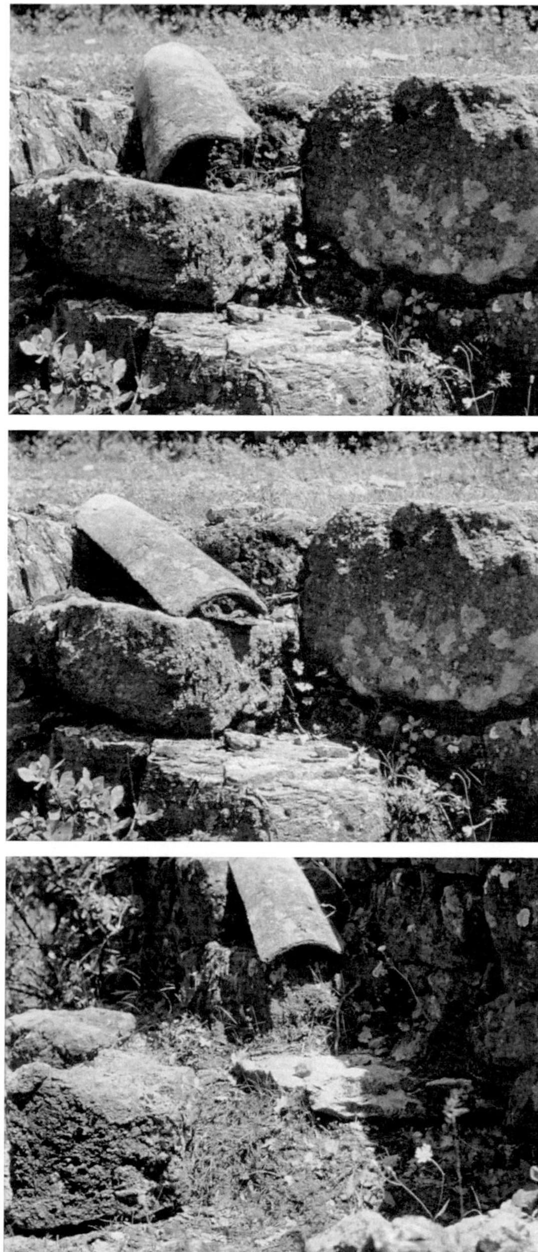

Animation sequence shot by Jacques Lin with a 35 mm camera, around 1982.

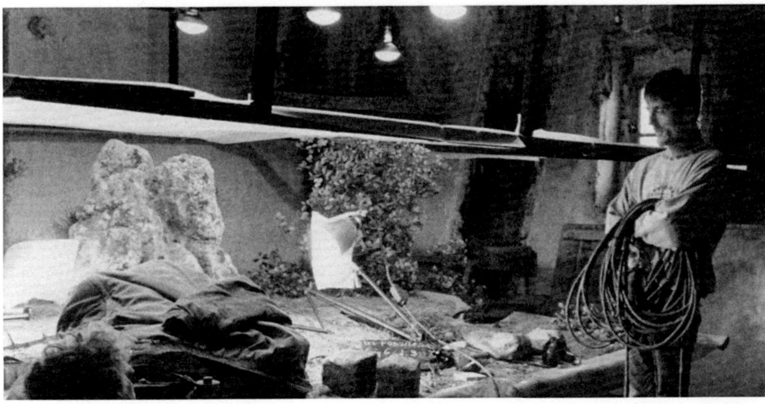

Gilles T. in the animation studio installed by Jacques Lin in the living area at Montplaisir, Monoblet, during shooting of the animated film *Les fossils ont la vie dure* (*Fossils Have a Hard Life*) in 1994.

Third, cameras were used to shoot the more consequential productions that played a role in giving the network visibility and presenting its experimental position, both clinically and ethically. *That Kid, There* (1975), in particular, which was directed by Renaud Victor and co-produced by Truffaut (Les Films du Carrosse), had a relatively large circulation and was often screened in clinical, educational, and cinephile contexts. This was also the case with *Projet N* [*Project U*, 1979 ('N' for 'Nous', 'Us')], which was directed by Alain Cazuc and produced by Thierry Garrel and the INA (French National Audiovisual Institute). These two documentaries took entirely different approaches to presenting life in the network: the first is black and white, very much a silent film,[73] and offers a sober, almost monastic, atmosphere; the second is colourful, and shows a more collective and even 'hippie' atmosphere. But the films have in common a preoccupation with presenting the very unique way of life in the network and are traversed by Deligny's poetic storytelling and reflections. Furthermore, both directors lived in the network for periods—they were part of it and not outsiders there solely to document it from an external perspective. In the years that followed, Victor became Deligny's main interlocutor when it came to cinema. With him, Deligny developed a sort of Socratic relationship and discussed movies,[74] concepts on the image, and film projects—among them several fictional works that were never finished;[75] Victor is the primary 'image taker', the virtual interlocutor mentioned in several texts published in this volume, some of which are even addressed to him. A few of these fictional projects were incorporated into the 1989 film *Fernand Deligny. À propos d'un film à faire* (*Fernand Deligny. About a film to make*), directed by Victor and co-produced by Bruno Muel[76]—the work was indeed a sort of conceptual *film to come*, mixing shots of these projects, a few scenes that had been staged, and

Deligny's readings and reflections on the image. Also of note is *Le faire et l'agir* (1979), directed by his daughter Caroline Deligny, and cut by a group of people associated with the University of Lyon. Unfortunately, its circulation was very limited. It was filmed with a Paluche video camera, which had recently been invented by Jean-Pierre Beauviala—and which would be used for example by Claude Lanzmann in his *Shoah*. Since the camera was very small, held by hand, and enabled a dissociation between the eye and the hand, entirely new perspectives were possible; Caroline Deligny, who spent some time in the network between 1977 and 1979, shot many hours of impressive and very sensitive images of the children, living areas, and elements of the landscape, particularly the water.

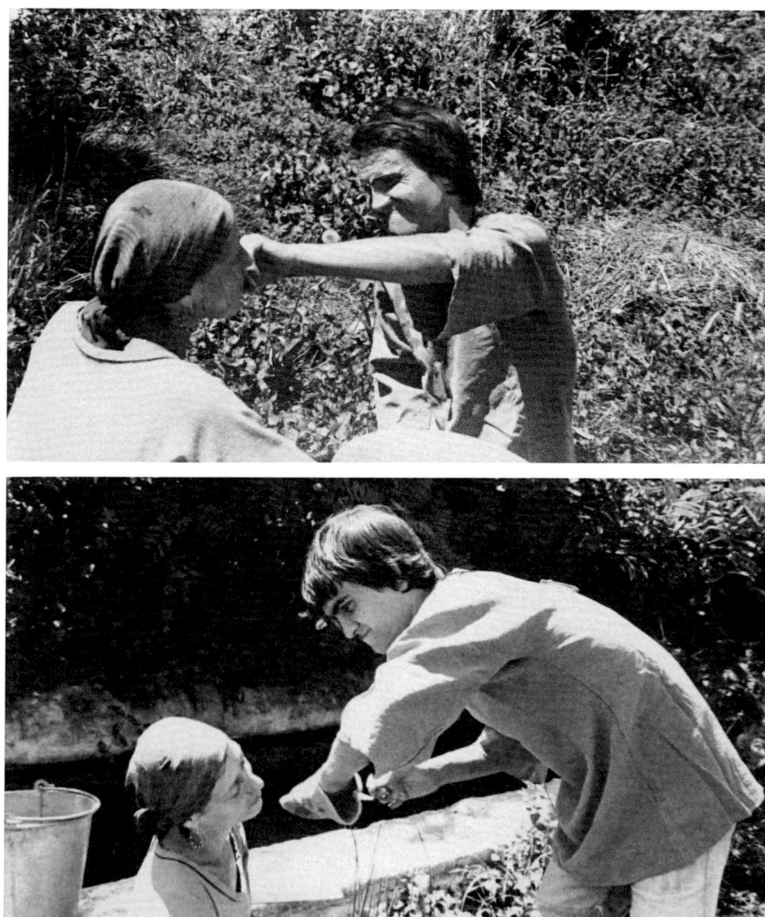

Gisèle Durand-Ruiz and Janmari during the shooting of *Project U*, directed by Alain Cazuc, 1978.

The turning point in Deligny's reflection in the late 1970s coincides with the first known occurrence of the neologism *camérer*, an infinitive in French,[77] which was precisely when Deligny's daughter began shooting with the Paluche. The term is the title of a series of texts, as was mentioned earlier, but is also used conceptually in many other pieces and in explicative remarks in the scripts. The use of the infinitive form—often translated as the gerund, 'camering', in this volume—recurs throughout Deligny's texts. It takes inspiration in the autistic children's form of 'acting' (*agir*), thus emphasising the action that is non-subjective and endless—in its double connotation of 'without goals' and 'ceaseless'. With 'camering', it is the cinema as a process that is highlighted: 'I maintain that camering doesn't come to an end and it's perhaps here that it differs from filming'.[78] Furthermore, as Deligny did twenty years prior in 'The Camera, a Pedagogical Tool', here he once again emphasises the tool—the camera—instead of the primacy of the object, the film. He believed that the camera should not be regarded mainly as an instrument that produced a finished object and he sought to demonstrate that the camera could 'make something quite different from a film'.[79] Indeed, most of his definitions of 'camering' are negative. In 'Miscreating', he emphasises that camering is an attempt 'to avoid intention' or that it is the 'the surfeit of intention', and that this requires 'a strange rigour that can't be intentional'.[80] If one wants to search for more positive definitions, one must look to the purpose of camering, its connection to the ideas of 'gathering' (*recueillir*) or 'catching' (*attraper*) images. From these provocative reflections, it follows, then, that the aim of camering is to achieve what Deligny feels the traditional form of filming seems generally incapable of, i.e., taking images.

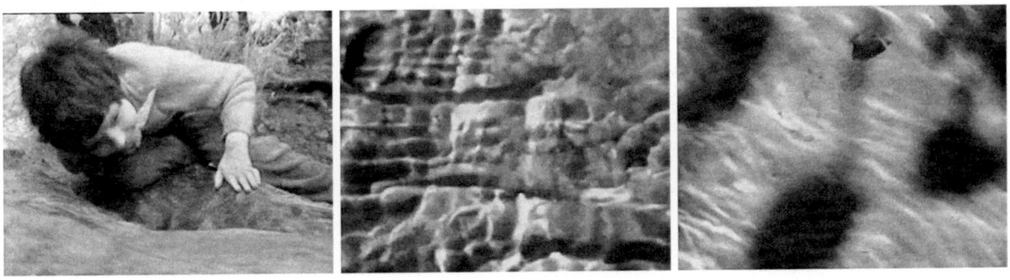

Images shot by Caroline Deligny with the Paluche Camera in the network, 1978-1979.

As we will see in detail, Deligny's reflection on camering is indissociable from his reconceptualisation of the notion of the 'image'. His proposition is to think of the image as being outside the reign of intentionality and subjectivity. For him, images can only appear 'by accident': they require a well-placed camera, and only then is it possible to gather them. That is why, beginning in 'Fossils Have a Hard Life: Apropos of the Image', he refers to the 'image taker' rather than the director, filmmaker, or any other of the terms traditionally used.

'Camering' is thus to be read as a conceptual and speculative term related both to a gesture—a form of practising—and a horizon—of experimentation. Its formulation also implies a completely different temporality from that of conventional shooting, as in a sense, it is emancipated from the commercial timeframe of production. In one of the 'Camering' pieces, Deligny associates the term with 'natural history', claiming to 'dream of camering the path of an iceberg and its thaw and the succession of changes in its appearance […] The event camered in real time, weeks would be needed to render it, to reproduce it; permanent cinema. Nothing but the iceberg on the screen for weeks'.[81] We saw that the idea of a 'permanent film' was already present during La Grande Cordée period. Here, however, it is the extended temporality of shooting that is emphasised—in a similar manner to that in Andy Warhol's early experimental films, such as *Sleep* (1964) and, in particular, *Empire* (1964).

In more practical terms, Deligny thus seems to think about cinema not through the goal (the film-product), but through its experimental dimension, where both time and integration into a specific space constitute its fundamental features. As with the living areas that hosted the autistic children, 'camering' requires that a 'customary' space be set up, one in which the camera becomes an integrated element of the installation, and is then capable of capturing images of the gestures, wanderings, moving bodies. Turning away from images that might signify or represent something—even if, in a sense, the aim is still to document (for example, Yves's gestures in *The Slightest Gesture* or those of Janmari in *That Kid, There*)—Deligny looks beyond the traditional documentary model for something that, from his perspective, could avoid forms of discursivity that *say* who the other is (that label, categorise, identify, signify); something that remains surprising and unknown; something open to the presence of materials, bodies, and gestures. In 'What Is Not Seen (by the Self)', a text that appeared several years later in *Cahiers du cinema* (1990) and is included in this volume,[82] Deligny defines the practice as 'ultra customary', as being both fiction and documentary, or, at the same time, neither: 'It's a genuine documentary. And for good reason: You can't get Janmari to do anything other than what he does every day. One couldn't make more of a documentary than that. And it makes the film a fictional work because folks have never experienced anything like it. It's neither documentary, nor fiction; it's the customary, this customary being so real that it surprises.'[83]

He felt that ultra-customary cinema would make visible what one is not used to, what perhaps remains unknown. Its function, I could add, is to 'puncture' representation. This theme runs through many of the texts in this volume. In 'Miscreating', Deligny insists on the 'disappointing' rather than the 'fulfilling' aspect of art, on the necessity of going beyond the 'mirage, each of us mirrored in it', of opening a 'breach whereby the human—that people are not at all conscious of—takes *forms*'.[84] And later, in the same text, he claims that 'it's a matter of putting out a new carbon copy of the same people as always, the viewer content as can be at recognising themself just as they were taught they are.'[85] Deligny's proposition is inscribed in a tradition of critiquing the film as an object of consumption.[86] With such film-objects, a subject is impelled to watch images that only project what is already known: ways of behaving, of feeling, of being in the world. The imagination is reactivated by objects that it already possesses. The subject accesses recognition-images, 'carbon copy' images (*copie conforme*, he writes, as in the title of one of Abbas Kiarostami's last films), which somehow confirm their convictions—and the diversity of human life forms is thus reduced to the one already-known vision of Mankind. In 'Miscreating', he insists: 'the film [is] a finished product destined to be delivered to the other's gaze, the other projecting their influence on the images to be taken, the sequences always/already taken in that inevitable cadastre of measured time, the representation always/already there, inevitable, in all that presented itself in the camera's frame.'[87]

This circular process of recognition and (re)production is at the very core of the narcissistic structure of subjectivity. That is why Deligny constantly emphasises the use of reflexive pronouns—something difficult to transpose into English—which is apparent in the original title of the 1990 text: *Ce qui ne* se *voit pas*. Something cannot be seen, in the first place, because of the all-encompassing presence of the subject (of the *se*, the 'self')—or rather, we should add, of a dominant, normalised, and major form of subjectivity that makes one say, for example, that an autistic child is deprived of 'normality'. Following his reasoning, subjects 'don't see anything' and in total opposition to this state of affairs, 'the task of cinema', the 'urgency of cinema is this: to revive that which among them is numbed, dazed, squandered, overnourished'.[88]

In 'Camering' (1982), the same questions appear in different formulations. Deligny takes over from Jean Epstein, a crucial theoretical and cinematographic reference for him, to think about this task, and relates it to the '"revolutionary power" of cinema', to its capacity as 'a privileged instrument that, like the telescope or the microscope, reveals aspects of the universe that were previously unknown'.[89] Contrary to filming, which shows known images that say what a person's body or gestures should be like, the aim of camering, Deligny feels, is to reveal something that has remained unknown because it is undermined by our general and established perception. Epstein praised the importance of chance, of coincidence, and argued that cinema was capable of producing a 'geography of gestures'.[90] In this geography, it was not the recognition of a certain gesture that he searched for, but rather stupefaction, and the oddness or uncanny nature of an unknown gesture. For Epstein, a certain use of the camera, of this 'eye outside the eye', would allow us to finally escape 'the tyranny of our egocentric and personal vision'.[91] This formulation matches up with a statement made by Deligny, in which he writes 'this other retina perceiving with another eye'.[92]

Indeed, Deligny often mentions the importance of chance in camering. In 'The Alga and the Fungus', a text on the collaborative relationship between he who writes and he who takes images—in French, *l'écrivant* ('the writor') and *le camérant* ('the cameror'), the use of the present participle again emphasising the processual dimension of the act—Deligny discusses shooting with the latter, Renaud Victor, and says: 'Treat chance as you do the light: with the utmost respect and even a bit of fear.'[93] If the 'writor' plays with words, the 'cameror' plays with the material of chance rather than that of image. In this sense, camering, as a practice willing to escape intentionality and self-reproduction, implies a *dispositive*, something that counters the director's drive of anticipating what they want to see and shoot, that helps them 'disintentionalising'.[94] That is why 'camering' involves the setting-up of a 'shooting area' (*aire de tournage*), a 'shooting dispositive' (*dispositif de tournage*),[95] that is integrated into customary life and enables, through its persistence, the shooting of unexpected, unanticipated images. For the same reason, Deligny prefers the word 'canvas' to that of script, as he describes in 'Fossils Have a Hard Life: Apropos of the Image'. He writes that one must create canvases 'that will lend themselves to coincidences'.[96] Different from a very defined playscript, the *canovaccio* in the *commedia dell'arte* is a support for improvisation, for the setting-up of situations. In French, the use of the term *canevas* in cinema is not unique to Deligny, but he takes it over precisely to emphasise this openness and its opposition to closed, intentional, and prescribed forms of scripts. He adds that the *canevas* does not constitute a perfect form, as it should be 'coarse' and full of 'holes'.[97] The holes constitute the favourable milieu that allows images to 'come through'.

Point of Seeing

These reflections and Deligny's insistence on the camera's potential can surely be misleading. However, it is noteworthy that he does not naively assume that the supposed objectivity of the camera will override the director's subjectivity, nor that the camera will enable a supposed total visibility.[98] His reflections are in fact very distant from models of permanent surveillance where observing-documenting takes place from the exterior. On the one hand, Deligny's proposition targets the personal point of view of the subject behind the camera, and the dangers of self-reproduction and self-projection; on the other hand, and this is crucial to understanding his position, he insists on the importance of the camera being *there*, operating within the living milieu as an integrated and customary element. The camera does not simply observe; it helps build the milieu from within. He writes that this 'entails the camera being *there* to so great an extent that it's the camerographer and their intentions and their point of view that fade before the point of seeing'.[99] It is not so much a question of recording as it is of keeping records, traces, documentation that, as already mentioned, aim at a multiplication of perspectives. This is what makes Deligny's notion of the 'point of seeing' (*point de voir*, in opposition to *point de vue*, 'point of view') so intriguing and a critical tool against the dangers of reducing reality to a single personal perspective. The point of seeing always concerns what is marginalised, what is 'refractory' to the dominant and conventional forms imposed by society.[100]

Though the notion first appeared in Deligny's vocabulary in 1976, it was in part developed and inspired by his exchanges with Robert Kramer, who visited him in the Cévennes in 1979. In a letter to Deligny, Kramer expresses his concern about 'camering' and the idea of 'an omniscient eye-camera' that would ideologically obliterate the 'subjectivity of the camera' and the fact that there is always a 'point of view'.[101] But in his response to Kramer, Deligny sticks to his position, and introduces a eulogy to the 'artifice' to help 'thwart the drive to represent oneself', which is important to counteract the effects of the 'dominant ideology'.[102] Also in his preparation notes for 'Miscreating', he argues that the 'artifice' makes it possible 'to glimpse the Real'.[103] As he often does in the texts written during this period, Deligny uses the Lacanian notion of the Real to refer to that which is outside the symbolic, the discourse, and thus resists attempts at signification. Following his argumentation, the dominant ideology has (a) language and the Real appears as what breaches this ideology, firstly, because it escapes language. Deligny's preoccupation here is, as always, to break with the usual representations of autism. To exemplify what he understands by 'artifice', he then describes how the camera can perceive a seed of wheat growing—time-lapse allows us to see what the human eye otherwise could not—and he asks if other artifices would not also be useful in exploring the human. The core of his argumentation is, once again, the following: 'It is necessary to leave our point of view, which is somewhat unanimous, in order to find a point of seeing, this point of seeing not being someone's. Hence the necessity of the artifice that will enable us to break, at least a little, the pact on which is based the man conscious of himself and through which this universal connivance is established'.[104]

The notion of a point of seeing is thus indissociable from an ethical horizon—Deligny takes the word 'ethics' from Wittgenstein and it becomes even more central in 'The Distinctiveness of the IMAGEs'—i.e., from the struggle against the universalisation of established conventions and the dominant ideology that determines how one is or should be. The invention of artifices that enable detours appear to Deligny as strategic forms to foil the inevitable reproductive dimension of the subjective gaze, to foil its 'convention arsenal'.[105]

Image(s)

For Deligny, a director is not truly concerned with the practice of image-taking if they pre-imagine their shots to too great an extent. Dazed by their own point of view, they remain in a state of auto-reproduction where the other always appears similar to them, a mere mirrored projection. For the image, as Deligny wants to conceptualise it, cannot be anticipated; on the contrary, the image is that which interrupts the subject's imagination. That is the reason behind the provocative statement he made in 1990; despite everything, he claims, 'We don't live in the age of the image', but instead in the era of 'verbalised reproduction'.[106]

The image as Deligny regards it is related to the Real and should evacuate the excess of subjectivism. It should at least be capable of 'stranging' the subject. In French, Deligny uses the infinitive form of the verb *étranger*. In English, the infinitive 'to strange', which is obsolete today, comes from the Latin *extraneus*, 'that which is on the outside'. The image, as conceptualised here, is precisely what comes from outside, what is unknown, uncanny, and strikes the interiority of the subject, their language, and their convictions.

When speculating on the image, Deligny makes a coupled conceptual distinction. On the one hand, some images are a reproduction of oneself and thus of a certain conception of Man, i.e., mirror, monumental, or, as he brilliantly puts it in 'Fossils Have a Hard Life: Apropos of the Image', 'iconic' images: 'the Man that we are has an image of himself, as it were, and this image is not distinctly speaking an image, but imagery, the product of naturalisation; Man is his own icon—the icon is incorporated'.[107] On the other hand, there exist images that are scraps (*lambeaux*) or full of 'holes':[108] 'images don't represent anything at all. That's why they're images; they themselves have no signification. Anyone who says sign, says code; you might as well tell wild geese to respect the Highway Code or the Air Traffic Code'.[109] Deligny relates these images both to the notion of the 'trace'—in opposition to that of the 'sign', since they do not signify anything—and to 'stirrings'—to the power they have of moving the spectator. In French, Deligny prefers the word *émoi* to dissociate it from its subjective and psychological dimensions, in a way that is close to Deleuze's use of the word 'affect'—one can speak of the *émoi* of bees or leaves, for example. In *Acheminement vers l'image* (*On the Way to the Image*), a text contemporary to 'Fossils Have a Hard Life: Apropos of the Image', Deligny further develops the motif of the wild geese in order to make a new, but analogous, distinction between 'domesticated' and 'consumable' images, on one side, and 'wild' or 'savage' images, on the other. Whereas the first are 'weighed down with meaning, symbolically fat, saturated with intensions', the latter appear again as speechless, empty of meaning, but capable of flying, and of interrupting recognition. 'The images cannot be imagined. [...] The imagined images are domesticated and they don't fly very far'.[110]

Here Deligny criticises a form of imagination that works by analogy and through associations that are always limited to one's own subjective repertoire. His struggle is against the fetishisation of a supposedly free faculty of imagination. That is why images cannot be imagined—again, he makes use of the reflexive form, *les images ne s'imaginent pas*, because the 'S' of the subject, the self, is present to too great an extent. 'As long as the image taker doesn't leave the self, s, e, l, f . . . there will be no image.'[111]

'Camering' is an attempt to gather, to shoot, what escapes 'us'. In *On the Way to the Image*, Deligny says that he may well be in search of lost images (*à la recherche des images perdues*, echoing of course Marcel Proust's oeuvre)—in search of the images that disappeared during montage, or even those that were never shot, maybe those that are *inmontables*, as Marker put it.[112] In 'Camering' (1978-1983), Deligny writes a new eulogy, this time to the 'leftovers',[113] to that which remains outside the director's intentionality and ends up being left behind. It is a eulogy to those images that were forever lost, that could not be seen because so much of the self was there.[114] In this sense, Deligny is against the iconic images that naturalise what Man is—and that by doing so 'reject' and 'eliminate' the real images, putting them *hors-champ*, 'out of frame';[115] what he calls the 'human' in fact refers to a sort of image of the imageless. It is something concrete (a singular child and their gestures, for example) but that, not being similar to oneself, is not suited to any known image, and only appears in ephemeral, 'meaningless', leftover images. This is indeed the paradox inside which Deligny develops his speculation on the notion of the image.

The motif of wild geese also leads Deligny to a disanthropomorphisation of the notion of the image, to an affirmation that the image is 'part of the animal kingdom'.[116] The notion would in reality be species-specific and not at all a privilege of Man—in his writings, Deligny often refers to beavers, spiders, and termites, and to the specific images originating in a 'memory of the species'[117] that guide their complex architectural structures. According to him, and in a very Nietzschean tone,[118] Man, with his 'overnourished', overloaded symbolic culture, should instead try to (re) learn to think in pictures, through images. There is of course no such thing as a return to a 'first nature'—nor is it even a question of 'first' or 'origin' in Deligny's texts. It is instead a question of acknowledging the intrinsic violence of civilising processes. Doing so involves the necessity to once again give space to everything Man has excluded from his framework of essential features that define himself and that are responsible for giving him a pre-eminent position above the rest of nature. In the centre of the civilising process, Deligny places speech itself. In the very epoch of *tout est langage* ('everything is language'), he prepares his rebellion, and insists on the impossibility of universally defining the human even if it is through a diverse notion of the symbolic—he prepares what seems a sort of 'goodbye to language' (as the title of Jean-Luc Godard's 2014 film also suggests), or at least to the unquestionable empire of symbolic, signifying, and verbal language.

Indeed, in the 'The Distinctiveness of the IMAGEs', the text of an obsessed writer searching for the image until his last days, Deligny develops the 'mode of thinking' that is constituted by the image, and which cannot be said by, or reduced to, language. He now writes 'IMAGEs', in capital letters, englobing in a certain sense all the qualities he has thus far attributed to the notion of the image: wild, autistic, scrap, sparkle, trace, fossil, beastly, hole, myriad. . . .He has Wittgenstein—'our friend WITT'—as a virtual interlocutor and insists on the specificity, distinctiveness, and precariousness of the image that is always in danger of being hunted down and driven out again. It is necessary, according to him, to give 'asylum'[119] to the image.

Deligny's late texts struggle with what would constitute the key and distinct aspects, *le propre*, of the image, and the fact that, paradoxically, he does not stop writing. And there is no resolution, no final decision, that puts an end to a struggle such as this. Sometimes he claims that '[l]anguage doesn't allow us to evoke IMAGEs'; at other times, he accepts the existence of a poetic language capable of evoking it: 'The image I evoke—the IMAGEs [...]'.[120] Interestingly, many of his late texts take a new form: they are of a fragmentary nature, are constituted by short, enigmatic sentences, and make use of the aphorism, and even the haiku. In sum, he experiments with forms that might be more immediately pictorial.

The undecidable quality of Deligny's writings is not unique to this period, but can be said of each of the texts included in this volume. Indeed, rather than offering a positive theory of the image or a cinematographic method, these texts, many of them highly speculative in nature, function to disorganise our structured convictions.

If Deligny's system is often organised through coupled terms (image and language, human and man, gesture and speech . . .), it is precisely to resist binary thought. He is instead interested in the transitions from one pole to the other; he never assumes a synthesis, but rather invokes the interminable negotiation that takes place inside the 'contradictory', the 'simultaneous presence of things'.[121] Therefore, it is no coincidence that the motifs of 'symbiosis' and 'lichen' are so important to him. Indeed, they confirm a strategy of undecidability. They speak both to collaboration or association (and 'not confusion'[122])—between writing and 'imaging'/'camering', between word and image—and to a structural impurity of reality. This impurity implies the coexistence of different life forms and the care one must take not to exterminate the others.

Notes

1 This reception is due mainly to the work of L'Arachnéen, the Paris-based publishing house that published a massive volume of his *Œuvres* in 2007 (and then reissued it in 2017), reuniting a collection of texts written over more than fifty years, accompanied by an important critical apparatus (ed. by Sandra Alvarez de Toledo). Since then, numerous volumes have been published and translated into various languages, in particular *L'Arachnéen et autres textes* (*The Arachnean and Other Texts*, trans. into English by Drew S. Burk and Catherine Porter, Minneapolis, University of Minnesota Press, 2013) and the bilingual *Cartes et lignes d'erre / Maps and Wander Lines*, Paris, L'Arachnéen, 2013.

2 Stored and open to the public at the Institut Mémoires de l'édition contemporaine (IMEC) in Caen, France. I was responsible—along with Noelle Resende and Marina Vidal-Naquet—for the classification and organisation of Deligny's written archives from his Cévennes period (1967–1996). An alternative and expanded version of this volume in French was put together by Sandra Alvarez de Toledo, Anaïs Masson, Marina Vidal-Naquet, and myself (Fernand Deligny, *Camérer. À propos d'images*, Paris, L'Arachnéen, 2021).

3 'For an *attempt* is closer to a work of art than to anything else' (Fernand Deligny, 'Card Taken and Map Traced' (1979) in *The Arachnean and Other Texts*, *op. cit.*, p. 151); 'an attempt is a political fact' ('Le Croire et le Craindre' (1978), in *Œuvres*, *op. cit.*, p. 1153, my translation).

4 'In 1944, I did indeed write that short book in which I spoke about the particular job [of educator]. But it is not mine' (Fernand Deligny, 'Le groupe et la demande: à propos de La Grande Cordée' (1967) in *Œuvres*, *op. cit.*, p. 425, my translation).

5 Fernand Deligny, *Lettres à un travailleur social* (1984–1985), Paris, L'Arachnéen, 2016, p. 76, my translation.

6 'Acheminement vers l'image', in *Camérer. À propos d'images*, *op. cit.*, p. 220, a shorter version (which was first published in the *Œuvres*) is available on the *Encontro Deligny* website, ed. by Maurício Rocha and Marlon Miguel, PUC-Rio, 2018, https://deligny.jur.puc-rio.br/index.php/livros-e-publicacoes/.

7 As for many of Deligny's generation, his experiences of war and fascism are crucial to understanding his trajectory. His first affiliation with the Communist Party dates from 1933 and reflects the necessity he felt to join the anti-fascist movements.

8 *Enfance inadaptée*, in French. The term was coined in occupied Vichy France and aimed at the institutional structuring of policies regarding deviant, 'abnormal' children and adolescents. Deligny, along with figures such as Henri Wallon, Louis Le Guillant, and Lucien Bonnafé—all of whom had close ties with the Communist Party—played an important role in debates on the definition of the term, particularly in the immediate post-war period. Against a biological definition of maladjustment, they directed their efforts towards politicising the discussions and trying to demonstrate the sociological foundations of deviancy. For further reading, see the two fundamental works of Michel Chauvière, *Enfance inadaptée: l'héritage de Vichy*, Paris, Les éditions ouvrières, 1980; and Pierre-François Moreau, *Fernand Deligny et les idéologies de l'enfance*, Paris, Éditions Retz, 1978.

9 See also Robert Castel, *La gestion des risques*, Paris: Les éditions de Minuit, 2011. The question of why youth suddenly became so central an issue can in part be explained by the context—the need for physical strength during the war and later to rebuild the country. It can be described as a moment of discovery by State apparatuses that saw young people as constituting important 'human capital' and that considered it more affordable to readapt them and turn them into a profitable workforce than to confine them. This 'discovery', however, demanded technicity. An increasingly technocratic discourse would thus evolve in the decades following the emergence of the concept of *enfance inadaptée* until its replacement by that of 'handicapped'.

10 Fernand Deligny, 'Les enfants ont des oreilles' (1948/1976) in *Œuvres*, *op. cit.*, p. 351.

11 Deligny's experimentation was in many aspects similar to that taking place during the same period at the Saint-Alban psychiatric hospital, the birthplace of institutional psychotherapy. There, the idea of disrupting the traditional relationship between doctor and patient was central to breaking the internal circuit of the psychiatric institution. To create a 'healing collectivity' that patients participated in was very important in François Tosquelles's programme, as was the idea of 'integrating madness into society' (in *Recherches*, No. 17, March 1975, p. 87, my translation). The work *outside* the hospital was, in Tosquelles and Lucien Bonnafé's perspective, as important as the work inside it. Therefore, they talked about a 'geo-psychiatry' that would involve the former patient being inserted into a 'human geography' outside the asylum where they would fit in and feel progressively more integrated, while continuing to receive assistance during the necessary healing period. Tosquelles, Bonnafé, and Deligny's perspectives had in common an emphasis on linking clinical and re-educational practices to social and familial environments, where the treatment process was not conceived as isolation, but rather as integration into the milieu. However, Deligny differed from Saint-Alban in that he did not align himself with psychoanalysis, nor did he intend to create a new model of psychiatry, and he would not take part in the anti-psychiatric movement. He intended instead to find breaches where he worked, so that the instituted space could be reorganised. He was always more interested in precarious moments that left space for something different to take place. For a history of institutional psychotherapy in English, see Camille Robcis, *Disalienation. Politics, Philosophy, and Radical Psychiatry in Postwar France*, Chicago, The University of Chicago Press, 2021.

12 In *Œuvres*, *op. cit.*, pp. 161–214. Also available online in *Encontro Deligny*, *op. cit.*

13 We do not know much about their collaboration during this period. What is known is that in early 1948, Deligny's text, *Le mystère de l'éducation populaire*, appeared in the journal *DOC*, created by Joseph Rovan and Marker, and that the latter published a short review on Deligny's *Les Vagabonds efficaces* a few months later. For their correspondence, see also Fernand Deligny, *Correspondance des Cévennes 1968–1996*, Paris, L'Arachnéen, 2018.

14 'Fossils Have a Hard Life', *infra*, p. 138; 'Camering' [1982], *infra*, p. 108.

15 'The Camera, a Pedagogical Tool', *infra*, p. 60. The notion of a 'milieu' was central to Deligny's reflection and remained so until his last texts. During this period, he takes it over from Wallon in particular, who showed its fundamental dimension to the formation of the individual (see his *De l'acte à la pensée*, Paris, Flammarion, 1942). Later, Deligny further enriched his reflection with that of ethologists such as Konrad Lorenz, Karl von Frisch, Henri Fabre, and Irenäus Eibl-Eibesfeldt—interestingly, there is no trace of his having read Jakob von Uexküll.

16 'The Camera, a Pedagogical Tool', *infra*, p. 60.

17 *Idem*.

18 On Makarenko, see my paper: 'The Product of Circumstances. Towards a Materialist and Situated Pedagogy', in *Materialism and Politics*, ed. by Bernardo Bianchi, Emilie Filion-Donato, Marlon Miguel, Ayşe Yuva, Berlin, ICI Berlin Press, 2021, https://doi.org/10.37050/ci-20_08.

19 Unpublished letter to Irène Lézine, March 24, 1956, my translation. Lézine was the secretary at La Grande Cordée, in addition to being affiliated with the Communist Party, a psychologist, a translator of authors such as Makarenko and Lev Vygotsky, and a very important interlocutor of Deligny during this period.

20 A passage in 'The Distinctiveness of the IMAGEs' implicitly refers to this atmosphere and to the position Deligny sought to take at La Borde: 'At one psychiatric institution, I established myself as the keeper of a greenhouse where anyone who wanted to could go and paint. I never would have guessed that so many

mentally ill people wished to paint. It's because painting was a decoy; in that greenhouse, ONE—everyone—had the absolute right to keep silent' (*infra*, p. 213).

21 Deligny maintains a 'critical proximity with the psychoanalyst [Jacques Lacan]', as Igor Krtolica and Guillaume Sibertin-Blanc put it in their paper 'The children estranged from language: Fernand Deligny, in his time, and against Lacan', in *Psychoanalysis and History*, vol. 21, No. 2, 2019, pp. 211–227. However, Deligny was not properly speaking 'in charge' of patients at La Borde, as the authors assert at the beginning of the paper, and he began the network for autistic children in 1967 (rather than in 1969). Furthermore, as noted above, the network was established from the start by Deligny alongside other individuals (the Durand sisters, Lin, and the Auberts). On the relationship between Deligny's work and Lacan, see also the chapter I dedicated to the subject in *À la marge et hors-champ. L'humain dans la pensée de Fernand Deligny*, Université Paris 8, 2016, pp. 449–470, https://www.theses.fr/2016PA080020.

22 See Fernand Deligny, *Correspondance des Cévennes 1968–1996*, *op. cit.*

23 Deligny, 'L'homme sans convictions' (1980), in *Œuvres*, *op. cit.*, annex of the 2017 reedition, pp. 1845–1854.

24 Deligny to Louis-Pierre Jouvenet, in Jean-Michel Caillot-Arthaud, Claude-Louis Chalaguier, Louis-Pierre Jouvenet, *Deligny: 50 ans d'asile*, Toulouse, Privat, 1988, p. 38. See also, *Lointain prochain. Les deux mémoires*, Paris, Fario, 2012, pp. 24–27; and *Mémoire d'asiles* (Unpublished, 1984, IMEC Archives, pp. 53–54); 'Fossils Have a Hard Life: Apropos of the Image', *infra*, pp. 125, 126, 159, 160. The passage is roughly the same in each of these versions. Deligny describes what can be read as a constitutive, inter-specific, and formative experience for him as a subject. When he was a child, he was walking by himself at a funfair in Lille and saw small monkeys inside a parrot cage. The monkeys looked at him, terrified, and he felt ashamed of his kind, of those who were 'similar' to him and responsible for imprisoning the monkeys. He writes that at that moment, he felt compelled to 'de-solidarise' himself with Man.

25 'the Man that we are has an image of himself', 'Fossils Have a Hard Life: Apropos of the Image', *infra*, p. 140.

26 'The Camera, a Pedagogical Tool', *infra*, p. 59. Dudley Andrew, in his article 'Malraux, Bazin, and the Gesture of Picasso' (in *Opening Bazin. Postwar Film Theory and Its Afterlife*, ed. Dudley Andrew with Hervé Joubert-Laurencin, Oxford, Oxford University Press, 2011, pp. 153–166), also insists on this point, particularly via a sentence by André Malraux—which Deligny himself quoted—on cinema's interest in serving as a means other than language of 'connecting the person to the world' [*Ibid.*, p. 162; see 'What Is Not Seen (by the Self)', *infra*, p. 238]. Andrew goes on to briefly analyse 'The Camera, a Pedagogical Tool' and compares it to Bazin's examination of Henri-George Clouzot's *The Mystery of Picasso* (1856).

27 La Grande Cordée Project Report sent to Louis Le Guillant, May 19, 1954, p. 4, my translation, in La Grande Cordée Archives. To date, these archives remain unpublished. They were compiled by Huguette Dumoulin and trusted to Daniel Terral.

28 'The authors of the film . . . ', 1955, La Grande Cordée Archives, my translation.

29 Unpublished letter to François Truffaut, June 18, 1960, my translation, in the archives of La Cinémathèque française.

30 An exception before the war was the Cinematographic Cooperative for Laic Schooling and the two films made in 1927 by Freinet (both titled *Les Élèves de Bar-sur-Loup au travail*), who emphasised the importance of the act of filmmaking [Freinet 1928 *apud* Henri Portier, 'De l'utilisation du film comme outil pédagogique à l'appropriation du cinéma par les élèves comme outil de creation', in D. Nourrisson and P. Jeunet (eds.), *Cinéma-école: aller-retour*, Université de Saint-Étienne, 2001, p. 118]. We can also mention the Ciné-Liberté Cooperative, created during the Front Populaire era, with the idea of bringing together technicians, workers, and artists to shoot activist films [cf. 'La coopérative Ciné-Liberté est créée' (1936) *apud* Valérie Vignaux, 'Ciné-Liberté ou l'autre cinéma du Front Populaire', in L. Creton and M. Marie (eds.), *Le Front populaire et le cinéma français*, No. 27, pp. 55–62]. After the war, a few initiatives sought to follow in the steps of Cine-Liberté and considered the possibility of creating a 'division of amateur filmmakers' ('La Fédération française des ciné-clubs', *Bulletin de l'IDHEC*, No. 3, July 1946, p. 16). In 1948, Bazin, who was Deligny's neighbour for a short period, also emphasised the necessity of 'cinematographic training workshops destined for educators' (*André Bazin. Écrits complets*, éd. Hervé Joubert-Laurencin, Paris, Macula, 2018, p. 446, my translation). However, no productions were made, and from 1945 onwards, the focus was mainly on the creation of a large network of cine-clubs, thanks to the initiative of names such as Georges Sadoul, Jean Painlevé, and Jacques Prévert. Their goal was to counterweight the presence of mass media and the emphasis was primarily on debate (cf. André Bazin, 'Le mouvement des ciné-clubs en France depuis la Libération', in *Ibid.*, pp. 429–433). See also Dudley Andrew, *André Bazin*, Oxford, Oxford University Press, 2013, in particular chapter 5, in which Andrew analyses this period, as well as the encounter between Bazin and Deligny.

31 In another letter to Truffaut (dated from 1958), Deligny wrote that Marker had been 'very tempted' to make a documentary on La Grande Cordée, but that in the end he unfortunately did not have the time (in Bernard Bastide (org.), 'Correspondance François Truffaut-Fernand Deligny', in *1895*, No. 42, 2004, https://journals.openedition.org/1895/281). Also of interest here is a film project Deligny conceived of during

this period. He emphasised that the idea was to document how 'the organisation is made', as well as the 'successive assemblies with the adolescents, the difficulties our organisation [*organism*] has to overcome. These gathering scenes should be shot in the facilities where they take place' ('Faire le film'. Letter to the friends of La Grande Cordée, January 24, 1956, La Grande Cordée Archives, my translation). The proposal is very close to those carried out years later by the Medvedkin Group inside factories.

32 La Grande Cordée Project Report, *op. cit.*, p. 13, my translation.

33 The word first appears in 1950, cf. 'La Grande Cordée (2)', in *Œuvres*, *op. cit.*, p. 413.

34 Michel Foucault, 'The confession of the Flesh', in *Power/Knowledge: Selected Interviews & Other Writings 1972–1977*, ed. by Colin Gordon, New York, Pantheon Books, 1980, pp. 195–196. This edition translates '*dispositif*' as 'apparatus'.

35 La Grande Cordée Project Report, *op. cit.*, p. 12, my translation.

36 'The Camera, a Pedagogical Tool', *infra*, p. 60.

37 *Ibid.* This viewpoint was commonplace at the time and voiced, for example, by a number of intellectuals connected with the Institute of Filmology (1948–1963). Though Deligny never associated himself with this circle, Wallon, the president of La Grande Cordée and a crucial reference for Deligny, was then an active collaborator with the institute and also acknowledged the 'universality of film' (Henri Wallon, 'L'enfant et le film', in *RIF* (*Revue internationale de filmologie*), No. 5, 1949, p. 21, my translation). The institute was created by Gilbert Cohen-Séat and brought together figures such as Étienne Souriau, Edgar Morin, and even Maurice Merleau-Ponty (see François Albera and Martin Lefebvre, 'La filmologie, de nouveau', in *Cinémas*, vol. 19, No. 2–3, 2009, https://www.erudit.org/fr/revues/cine/2009-v19-n2-3-cine3099/).

38 'The Camera, a Pedagogical Tool', *infra*, p. 58.

39 *Idem.*

40 One finds echoes here of several reflections that immediately precede or are contemporary to those of Deligny. The problem of cinema as a natural or total reproduction of reality was largely developed by André Bazin (see in particular 'Le mythe du cinéma total' (1946), in *Écrits complets*, *op. cit.*, pp. 2557–2560). The revolutionary necessity of producing materials such as images and writings by oneself, and of teaching peers these techniques was central to Walter Benjamin (see in particular, 'The Author as Producer', in *New Left Review*, No. I/62, July-August 1970, https://www.marxists.org/reference/archive/benjamin/1970/author-producer.htm). Finally, in a sense, we can affirm that Aleksandr Medvedkin was the direct predecessor to Deligny. With his Kino-Train, Medvedkin aimed at making interventional and local productions that were immersed in a specific territory—'the production of a film is organically and intrinsically linked to its screening in the place of production' (Medvedkin *apud* Emma Widdis, *Alexander Medvedkin*, London, I.B. Tauris, 2005, p. 25); the Kino-Train films were 'helpful to us in interventions into crucial problems of those grim years—food, living conditions, physical and emotional well-being . . . ' (Medvedkin, 'The Kino-Train: 294 Days on Wheels', in *The Alexander Medvedkin Reader*, Chicago, The University of Chicago Press, 2016, p. 36). All in all, we can say that Deligny's discourse updates those of Benjamin and Medvedkin, which are to be read in the context of 'cinefication' (Cf. Pavlev Levi, *Cinema by other means*, Oxford, Oxford University Press, 2012), where the pursuit of the revolution, the transformation of society towards socialism, education, the seizure of power by the masses, and the fight for hegemony were indissociable from the massive investment in apparatuses and techniques, from the utopia of equipping the people with tools of representation.

41 'The Camera, a Pedagogical Tool', *infra*, p. 60.

42 'Le Ciné-Œil, le Radio-Œil et le soi-disant "documentalisme"', in *Dziga Vertov. Le Ciné-Œil de la révolution. Écrits sur le cinéma*, Paris, Les presses du réel, 2018, p. 400, my translation.

43 'Un chef d'œuvre du cinéma à faire' (Unpublished letter to Irène Lézine, April 1, 1955); 'The film was there, ready to be made' ('The Camera, a Pedagogical Tool', *infra*, p. 59); 'Faire le film'. Letter to the friends of La Grande Cordée, January 24, 1956, La Grande Cordée Archives.

44 The term does not appear in 'The Camera, a Pedagogical Tool', but it is recurrent in the other documents of this period: 'This "production"—a permanent documentary from which some shots could be cut and transformed into a presentable film' (Unpublished letter to Irène Lézine, March 12, 1955, my translation); 'This film, this permanent documentary' (Unpublished letter to Alexis Danan, July 1955, in La Grande Cordée Archives, my translation); a 'film being permanently shot' (*film qui se tourne en permanence*, 'The authors of the film . . . ', 1955, in La Grande Cordée Archives, my translation).

45 'We maintain that imperfect cinema must above all show the process which generates the problems. It is thus the opposite of a cinema principally dedicated to celebrating results, the opposite of a self-sufficient and contemplative cinema, the opposite of a cinema which "beautifully illustrates" ideas or concepts which we already possess' (Julio García Espinosa, 'For an imperfect cinema', translated by Julianne Burton, in *Jump Cut*, No. 20, 1979, pp. 24–26, https://www.ejumpcut.org/archive/onlinessays/JC20folder/ImperfectCinema.html). Espinosa's manifesto is written in the context of international recognition of Latin American cinema and it tackles the problem of *who* takes part in the cinematographic production process, *from where*, and according to which *forms*; it envisions production from the *periphery*, made by the *marginal*.

46 Indeed, referring to a discussion with Renaud Victor about La Grande Cordée, Deligny uses the formula 'to make a movie without film' ('The Distinctiveness of the IMAGEs', *infra*, p. 180). It is impossible not to think of Lev Kuleshov, who found himself in a similarly precarious position in terms of materials, and along with his collaborators began to stage 'films/movies without film' (*Fil'my bez plenki*). These were theatrical performances of sorts that were presented before a camera and that followed the principle of montage (cf. *Kuleshov on Film. Writings of Lev Kuleshov*, Berkeley, University of California, 1975, in particular the introduction and the chapter 'Our first experiences').

47 For a further analysis of these themes and period, see my essay 'Mettre la vie en œuvre: autour de "La caméra outil pédagogique"', in *Camérer. À propos d'images*, *op. cit.*, pp. 341–348.

48 'The speeches would be the music of the film and be treated as musical material' (Letter from Deligny to Truffaut, October 8, 1959, in *1895*, *op. cit.*, my translation).

49 *The Slightest Gesture* was produced by SLON (which later became ISKRA), a cooperative created by, among others, Marker. SLON is an acronym for Société pour le lancement des œuvres nouvelles (Society for Launching New Works) and additionally means 'elephant' in Russian, a reference to Alexander Medvedkin. The cooperative also produced the Medvedkin Group films.

50 Before entering the 'story', the film begins with a presentation of sorts in which Deligny asks, 'Why should the speech belong to someone even if this someone is speaking?' (*Pourquoi faudrait-il que la parole appartienne à quelqu'un, même si ce quelqu'un la prend ?*), in *Œuvres*, *op. cit.*, p. 608, my translation.

51 Gilles Deleuze, *The Time-Image*, London, The Athlone Press, 2000, pp. 183–184. Deleuze refers thereafter to Jean-Luc Godard in his 'erasure of the internal monologue as whole of the film in favour of a free indirect discourse and vision; the erasure of the unity of man and the world, in favour of a break which now leaves us with only a belief in this world' (*Ibid.*, p. 188). Also, Jacques Rancière, commenting on Godard's *La Chinoise*, emphasises the importance of the dissociation of word and image, the division 'in two of the One of the representative magma: to separate words and images, to make perceptible the strangeness of the words and the foolishness of the images' (*La Fable cinématographique*, Paris, Seuil, 2001, p. 190, my translation).

52 'He's Still One of Us', *infra*, p. 64.

53 Jean-Pierre Faye, *Langages totalitaires. Critique de la raison / de l'économie narrative*, Paris, Hermann, 2004, p. 4. See also his *Le langage meurtrier*, Paris, Hermann, 1996. Both in 'Fossils Have a Hard Life: Apropos of the Image' and 'The Distinctiveness of the IMAGEs', Deligny also associates language with the tyrant, and, inspired by La Boétie's reflection on 'voluntary servitude', he tries to deflate language and to think of a means of resistance against it: 'Language can undoubtedly be voted on. It's a tyrant with a good reputation. We sometimes speak about the power of words. Like the tyrant, language only ever has the power that is given to it—by its subjects. Certainly, and without doubt, language can say: it can say that it exists, it can also say that one has to say' (*infra*, p. 211).

54 Cf. Colette Soler, *L'inconscient à ciel ouvert*, Toulouse, Presse Universitaires du Mirail, 2012. In the voice-over text he wrote to accompany the images of *That Kid, There*, Deligny returns to the motif associating the roofless (*sans toit*) with the absence of the other (*sans toi*)—see 'Ce Gamin, là', in *Œuvres*, *op. cit.*, p. 1052; and 'Nous et l'Innocent', in *Ibid.*, p. 725. Regarding *The Slightest Gesture*, Deligny writes the following in 'The Distinctiveness of the IMAGEs': 'I made a feature film in which the hero was a knot' (*infra*, p. 192).

55 In the sense given by Georges Canguilhem, i.e., the immanent norms corresponding to each individual (see *The Normal and the Pathological*, Princeton, Zone Books, 1991). By considering autism as another 'mode of being', Deligny's proposition is indeed a radical one and certainly anticipates some of the debates in what is today termed 'neurodiversity'—see for example *The Minor Gesture* (Durham, Duke University Press, 2016) by Erin Manning, who writes: 'Neurodiversity is the path I choose here to explore insurgent life' (p. 5). In spite of the title, Manning does not mention Deligny in the book, though she does refer to him in her earlier work (*Always More Than One*, Durham, Duke University Press, 2012, chapter 8). Other contemporary practitioners and thinkers also propose viewing autism as a distinct 'structure', one that differs from schizophrenia and psychosis (see, for example, Jean-Claude Maleval 'Pourquoi l'hypothèse d'une structure autistique? (ii)', in *La Cause du Désir*, No. 88, pp. 153–164, 2014, https://doi.org/10.3917/lcdd.088.0153).

56 It is not surprising, then, that many readers of Spinoza in France were immediately drawn to Deligny's reflection, beginning, of course, with Deleuze, though we can also mention Pierre-François Moreau, who wrote the first monography on Deligny in 1978 (*Fernand Deligny et les idéologies de l'enfance*, *op. cit.*), and who has recently returned to his work (see in particular the volume Moreau co-edited with Michael Pouteyo, *Deligny et la Philosophie*, Lyon, ENS, 2021), Pierre Macherey (see, for example, *Le sujet des normes*, Paris, Les éditions Amsterdam, 2014, and the postface for *Lettres à un travailleur social*, *op. cit.*), and Pascal Sévérac (see, for example, 'L'agir au lieu de l'esprit', in *Intellectica*, 2012/1, No. 57, pp. 253–268, republished in Marlon Miguel and Maurício Rocha (eds.), *Cadernos Deligny*, Rio de Janeiro, PUC-Rio, 2018, https://cadernosdeligny.jur.puc-rio.br/index.php/CadernosDeligny). Spinoza's reflection on the perfectibility of each singular body and his critique on the notions of 'analogy' and 'privation' are well known. In his famous Letter 21 to Blijenbergh, the Dutch philosopher claims that one can only say that a blind man is deprived of something

(here his sight) as the effect of an impossible and thus imaginary analogy between two singular beings (cf. *The Collected Works of Spinoza*, ed. and trans. by Edwin Curley, vol. 1, Princeton, NJ, Princeton University Press, 1985, pp. 375–382).

57 Deligny refers, in the first place, to Claude Lévi-Strauss to think about the diversity of 'life forms' ('Les Détours de l'agir ou le Moindre geste' (1979), in *Œuvres, op. cit.*, pp. 1272–1274, where he quotes excerpts from an interview with the anthropologist, 'On m'a souvent reproché d'être antihumaniste', January 21–22, 1979, in *Le Monde*). We can also consider the famous chapter on 'The Archaic Illusion', in *The Elementary Structures of Kinship* (Boston, Beacon Press, 1971), in which Lévi-Strauss develops the idea of 'a common basis of mental structures and schemes' (p. 85) that is very diverse but will be the aim of a selective operation by a certain culture. Deligny is, of course, more interested in emphasising that this 'virtual' diverse 'substructure' (*soubassement*) remains present and active as a sort of *stratum*. His other reference to the reflection on stratification and fossilisation is André Leroi-Gourhan, in particular, *Gesture and Speech*, Cambridge, MA, MIT, 1993.

58 'We have to suppose—out of our own concern for seeing them as similar [*de les semblabiliser*], a concern that certainly comes from good intentions [...]. And we make a gift to the other of our own intention, so great is our generosity with respect to him or her. Once again we discover the image of human beings [the image of the Man] that is supposedly the same for one and all' (*The Arachnean and Other Texts, op. cit.*, p. 167). See also 'Miscreating', where camering and the whole 'attempt' appear as an effort to 'evade our inclination to similarise the other, whether or not they be autistic' (*infra*, p. 84).

59 'One eye + closer + closer / one no longer knows what it is / one is lost (finally / this one colonises us / everyone / and prevents us from seeing, from inventing, from divining / *for one knows the name of things*' ('*un œil + près + près / on ne sait plus ce que c'est / on est perdu / enfin / cet on qui nous colonise / chacun / et nous empêche de voir, d'inventer, de deviner* / parce qu'il sait le nom des choses'), 'Repères', unpublished, circa 1971, my translation). It is also interesting to note how Deligny, following a comment by Ivan Illich, associates Christopher Columbus's discovery enterprise with the project of imposing 'a maternal grammar as the language of the state' (*The Arachnean and Other Texts, op. cit.*, p. 104). In this sense, the colonisation process is indissociable from the institution of a 'major' language.

60 In *Œuvres, op. cit.*, p. 700, my translation.

61 *Ibid.*, p. 691, my translation.

62 Letter to Althusser, September 1976, in *Correspondance des Cévennes 1968–1996, op. cit.*, p. 565, my translation.

63 'Cahiers de l'immuable / 1', in *Œuvres, op. cit.*, pp. 847–848, my translation. The *Cahiers de l'Immuable* (The Notebooks of the Immutable) are a series of three volumes (a forth was planned and begun but never finished) that compile texts, documents, and images produced by Deligny, the close presences, and different collaborators and interlocutors involved with the network. They were published in 1975–1976 as separate volumes of the *Revue Recherches*, created by Guattari.

64 For more on the maps see, *Cartes et lignes d'erre / Maps and Wander Lines, op. cit.*

65 Despite this and the fact that another important word in Deligny's vocabulary is the *dérive* (drift), his approach is far from a romanticisation of the children's movements and is also very distant from the 'psychogeography' developed by the Situationists.

66 Deligny and his collective perceived what they call the importance of the 'immutable' (*immutable*)—which of course resonates with Leo Kanner's first definitions of autism in 1943 through his ideas of 'sameness' (*immutabilité*) and 'aloneness', but also shifts them, since the *immutable* is not conceived as total unchangeability. It is now known that autistic persons have an acute sensibility, a permeability to the environment, a 'sensory openness which is experienced as a bombardment of sensa' (Donald Meltzer, 'The Psychology of Autistic States and of Post-Autistic Mentality', in Donald Meltzer, John Bremner, Shirley Hoxter, Doreen Weddel, Isca Wittenberg, *Explorations in Autism. A Psycho-analytical Study*, Scotland, Clunie Press, 1975, p. 20). See also the descriptions by Temple Grandin, an autistic person, in her *Thinking in Pictures*, London, Bloomsbury, 2006. She claims that her stereotypies such as 'rocking' and 'spinning' were reactions whenever she felt 'overloaded' (p. 34) by perception. Interestingly, Deligny also often refers to autistic perception as 'thinking in pictures'.

67 'The distant and the close', *lointain prochain*, is also the title of a trilogy of texts by Deligny. Jean Oury, who wrote a good deal on this particular mode of 'proximity', might have been one of Deligny's interlocutors, and as was mentioned earlier, they did indeed spend time side by side at La Borde. Oury also reflects on these dialectics and claims that 'the greater proximity is to assume the distance of the other. This gives a sort of definition of the transference' (Jean Oury, 'Utopie, atopie et eutopie', in *Revue Chimères*, No. 28, Spring-Summer 1996, p. 75).

68 Deleuze perceived precisely how, on the one hand, the cartography developed in the network did not aim at 'interpreting' the children's behaviours ('What Children Say', in *Essays Critical and Clinical*, New York, Verso, 1998) and on the other, how it implied a form of 'performance' rather than revealing pre-given knowledge (Gilles Deleuze and Félix Guattari, 'Rhizome', in *A Thousand Plateaus: Capitalism and Schizophre-*

nia, Minneapolis, University of Minnesota Press, 2005, p. 12). Unfortunately, Deleuze and Guattari do not really analyse the cartographies in detail and surely the best text written during this period on the subject is that by Françoise Bonardel for an exhibition at the Centre Georges Pompidou in which some of the cartographies were displayed. As she writes, 'the "person" can no longer be designated by what they are (name, personality, intellectual aptitude reduced to nothing by psychosis), but by that which "takes place" through them. We watch the remarkable replacement of the usual and here ineffective psychology by a topography and topology' ('Lignes d'erre', in Giulio Macchi and Jacques Mullender (curators), *Cartes et figures de la Terre*. Exhibition Catalogue, Centre Georges Pompidou, May 24–November 17, 1980, p. 194, my translation).

69 This perspectivism does not of course mean putting oneself in the standpoint of the other. One can think here of Eduardo Viveiros de Castros and his reflections on the anthropological work he has carried out and on the notion of perspectivism: 'What I did in my article on perspectivism was a thought experiment and an exercise in fictional anthropology. The expression 'thought experiment' does not have the usual meaning of accessing the imaginary in an experience through one's (own) thought, but rather of accessing the (other's) thought through the real experience: it is not a question of imagining an experience, but of experimenting an imagination. In this case, the experience is mine as an ethnographer and a reader of an ethnological bibliography on indigenous Amazonia, and the experimentation is a fiction controlled by this experience. That means that the fiction is anthropological, but its anthropology is not fictive' (Eduardo Viveiros de Castro, 'O nativo relativo', *Mana*, vol. 8, No. 1, 2002, p. 123, my translation). The ideas of a 'thought experiment' and an 'imagined experiment' are taken from Ludwig Wittgenstein (*Philosophical Remarks*, Oxford, Blackwell, 1998, p. 52; and *Philosophical Investigations*, §265, Oxford, Blackwell, 1986, p. 94e), who was also an important reference for Deligny in his later years and is quoted in some of the texts included in this volume.

70 Deligny claims he is the 'storyteller rather than the leader' (*le conteur plutôt que le meneur*) of the different 'approaches and attempts' in which he engaged himself ('Des réseaux et des hommes', in *Revue Mêlée*, Nimes / Marseille, Offset avenir, No. 2, November 1981, p. 10, my translation).

71 It is also worth mentioning that Deligny was against his name appearing on the cover, but finally agreed as a result of Guattari's insistence. For a reflection (and critique) of the author's name, see his 'L'homme sans convictions', in *Œuvres*, *op. cit.*, pp. 1845–1854.

72 This is the case with Lin's recent *Aucun d'eux ne dit mot* ('None of them says a word'), in which he presents later images of the work continued by himself and another close presence, Gisèle Durand. The film was screened for the first time in 2020 at the *Cinéma du Réel* festival. It was produced by Richard Copans (Les Films d'ici), who also worked with Victor and Deligny, and recently directed the more commercial documentary *Monsieur Deligny, vagabond efficace* (2019). Lin is additionally the author of *La vie de radeau* (Marseille, Le mot et le reste, 1996/2007), a crucial account of life with the autistic persons in the network.

73 The silence is very much inhabited and the many sounds one hears of everyday life and elements of the landscape are a crucial aspect of the film. It is 'a rich, living silence' as Marguerite Duras said of her own films ('Cinema', in *The Suspended Passion*, London, Seagull Books, 2016). A few lines later, she affirms: 'the reality reproduced by classical cinema has never been of any interest to me'. Indeed, many connections can be made between Marguerite Duras's thoughts on the practice and role of writing about/on cinema and those of Deligny. They offer similar and interesting reflections on the ways in which the image and words can collaborate. 'It was as though the word I wrote already contained its image within itself. To film it was to pursue the discourse and amplify it. It was to continue writing—on the image' (*Idem*).

74 It is difficult to state precisely which movies served as references for Deligny. One does know that he was fond of experimental European avant-garde works such as those by Man Ray and Walter Ruttmann—*The Starfish* (1928) and *In der Nacht* (1931) are cited by him in the first text in this volume; Soviet productions, including *Storm Over Asia* (Vsevolod Pudovkin, 1928), which was screened many times by the adolescents of La Grande Cordée, and *Road to Life* (Nikolai Ekk, 1931), mentioned in a few of the texts published here; *The Threepenny Opera* (G. W. Pabst, 1932), and the films of Jean Epstein. It is also known that Deligny (with Lin) screened movies at La Borde on the Vietnam War, such as Wilfred Burchett's *Maquis Viet Cong* (1965). During this time, he met Jean Renoir at the clinic; Renoir had watched, and liked, according to Deligny, some of the rushes from *The Slightest Gesture*. Deligny also mentions Jean Rouch—prior to seeing his films—as an inspiration for *The Slightest Gesture*; Czech animation films, possibly those by Karel Zeman; and Herbert J. Biberman's *Salt of the Earth* (1954).

75 Deligny wrote many 'scripts', particularly in the 1980s. Most of them remain unpublished and are stored at the IMEC. They are curious in that they fall somewhere between true scripts, novels, and long synopses; they often have several variations and in general are quite repetitive and would be difficult to publish as such. Among the numerous pieces Deligny wrote, we can mention, for example, *Peaux d'argile* (Clay skin), a sort of fable of beings who live inside a cave and their encounter with a young boy from the Cévennes. The

director Fernand Moskowicz showed interest in filming *Peaux d'argile* and a version of the manuscript includes a short text by him. Other works of note are *Toits d'asiles* (Asylum rooftops), which Renaud Victor had planned to direct, and which addresses the rumours around and disappearance of a Brazilian boy living in Graniers—some shots of the film can be seen in *Fernand Deligny. À propos d'un film à faire* (*Fernand Deligny. About a film to make*, 1989); and *Rue de l'Oural*, a fictional piece written in 1981 about the post-war period in Paris, which takes place in an occupied theatre.

76 Who directed, among other films, *Week-end à Sochaux* (1972), in the context of the Medvedkin Group.

77 Letter to Isaac Joseph, March 3, 1977, in *Correspondance des Cévennes*, *op. cit.*, p. 648.

78 'Camering' [1978], *infra*, p. 74.

79 'Camering' [1978–1983], *infra*, p. 165.

80 'Miscreating', *infra*, p. 83.

81 'Camering' [1978–1983], *infra*, p. 167.

82 The text is in fact the compilation of extracts from an interview by Renaud Victor and Serge Le Péron. Numerous conversations between Victor and Deligny took place during this period and are stored in the archives at the IMEC.

83 'What Is Not Seen (by the Self)', *infra*, p. 237.

84 'Miscreating', *infra*, p. 78.

85 *Ibid.*, p. 84.

86 He is even clearer on this in one of the 'Camering' texts: 'Projections are consumer goods. Thus functions a recovery circuit in which household rubbish holds on tight to what's imagined, projected' ['Camering' [1978], *infra*, p. 69]. In another text, he criticises the cinema as a spectacle, and again its provision of ready-made images for the viewer. 'The work resulting from "camering" is in fact not a spectacle. It is instead an attempt in which the "viewers" are invited, impelled, to take part. [...] ONE proposes—imposes—cars, travels to Singapore, HI-FI audio systems [...] Folks are served [*servis*]—enslaved [*asservis*]. [...] They must be provided with ready-to-see [*prêt-à-voir*]—as one would say ready-to-wear [*prêt-à-porter*]' (Notes on *A Better Life*, p. 6, unpublished, circa 1985, in IMEC Archives).

87 'Miscreating', *infra*, p. 85.

88 'What Is Not Seen (by the Self)', *infra*, p. 237.

89 'Camering [1982]', *infra*, p. 106.

90 Jean Epstein, *Écrits sur le cinéma*, Tome 1, *L'objectif lui-même*, p. 128, my translation.

91 *Idem*, p. 129.

92 'Acheminement vers l'image', in *Camérer. À propos d'images*, *op. cit.*, p. 189, my translation.

93 'The Alga and the Fungus', *infra*, p. 117. The symbiosis motif also appears in 'The Distinctiveness of the IMAGEs', *infra*, p. 173.

94 'What Is Not Seen (by the Self)', *infra*, p. 236.

95 'Miscreating', *infra*, p. 84; 'Acheminement vers l'image', in *Camérer. À propos d'images*, *op. cit.*, p. 206.

96 'Fossils Have a Hard Life: Apropos of the Image', *infra*, p. 129.

97 *Idem.*

98 It is for this reason that Deligny's reflection is to be inscribed in the avant-garde tradition of Epstein or Vertov rather than that of Harun Farocki, who largely developed the question of visibility (the word appears for example in the original title of his 1981 *Etwas wird sichtbar / Before Your Eyes Vietnam*). For Deligny, the camera conceived of as a tool is indeed a prosthesis, an extension of the human, rather than its substitution. 'Farocki intimates that a new "robo eye" is in place, one that, unlike the "kino eye" celebrated by modernists like Dziga Vertov, does not extend the human prosthetically so much as it replaces the human robotically' (Hal Foster, 'Vision Quest: The Cinema of Harun Farocki', in *Artforum*, November 2004, p. 160).

99 'Miscreating', *infra*, p. 98.

100 'In a given "milieu", there is what we see from us—regarding us and from our point of view—and, implicitly [*en filigrane*], appears what is spotted from the point of seeing of an individual, and is refractory to what the environing society has proposed and imposed in terms of what they acquire and are. [...] There is the "point of view" and there is the "point of seeing" that is refractory to the formulable' ('Atelier INA', in *Camérer. À propos d'images*, *op. cit.*, p. 45, my translation).

101 Robert Kramer, Letter to Deligny, May 30, 1979, in *Correspondances des Cévennes*, *op. cit.*, p. 873.

102 Deligny, Letter to Kramer, in *Ibid.*, p. 876.

103 'Notes pour "Mécréer"', in *Camérer. À propos d'images*, *op. cit.*, p. 72, my translation.

104 *Idem.*

105 'Fossils Have a Hard Life', alternative version, in *Camérer. À propos d'images*, *op. cit.*, p. 143, p. 146 and 'Acheminement vers l'image', in *Ibid.*, pp. 167–168. According to Deligny, the term was taken from Néstor Almendros. Deligny relates an interesting reading of the cinematographer's obsession with natural light.

He does not see it as a sort of naturalism, but on the contrary, as an artifice that ends up artificially imposing a longer temporality on shooting. One has to wait for the perfect light, and this opens the space to time and thus to chance. It is the introduction of such detours that, according to Deligny, provide the occasion to perhaps shoot in a different manner.

106 'What Is Not Seen (by the Self)', *infra*, p. 235.

107 'Fossils Have a Hard Life: Apropos of the Image', *infra*, p. 140. One can think here of a similar reflection by Einstein, quoted by Isabelle Stengers and Ilya Prigogine in their 1984 book that was almost contemporary to Deligny's text (1982): 'Man seeks to form for himself, in whatever manner is suitable for him, a simplified and lucid image of the world (*Bild der Welt*), and so to overcome the world of experience by striving to replace it to some extent by this image', Albert Einstein, 'Prinzipien der Forschung, Rede zur 60. Geburtsag van Max Planck' (1918) *apud* Isabelle Stengers and Ilya Prigogine, *Order out of chaos*, London, Verso, 1984/2017, Introduction, section 5.

108 In a letter to Claude Chalaguier (May 6, 1988) written during the same period as 'The Distinctiveness of the IMAGEs', one finds: 'I have recently realised that ONE uses the word image to plug the hole, because language has a hole; the word image is the hole' (in *Correspondance des Cévennes, op. cit.*, p. 1143, my translation).

109 'Fossils Have a Hard Life: Apropos of the Image', *infra*, p. 141.

110 'Acheminement vers l'image', in *Camérer. À propos d'images, op. cit.*, pp. 1667–1671, my translation. This text was also written in 1982, likely just after 'Fossils Have a Hard Life: Apropos of the Image' (and its alternative version 'Fossils Have a Hard Life'). Since it is quite long and in many aspects similar to the latter, the decision was made not to include it in this volume, despite its importance.

111 'What Is Not Seen (by the Self)', *infra*, p. 236. See also the short aphorism in 'The Distinctiveness of the IMAGEs', where he claims that 'The imaginary [...] has nothing to do with the IMAGEs' (*infra*, p. 202).

112 Marker begins *Sans Soleil* (1983) with the idea of a non-editable image, an impossible image that 'cannot associate itself with other images'; he finishes it with 'these images already affected by the lichen of the Time' ('Sans soleil', in *Trafic*, No. 6, 1993, p. 79 and p. 96). The lichen is also a recurrent motif in Deligny's writing.

113 'Camering' [1978–1983], *infra*, p. 169.

114 João Moreira Salles in his film *Santiago* (2007) quotes Werner Herzog to claim that the most important thing in cinema is probably that which is 'leftover'. Indeed, Salles's film was made of material filmed thirteen years prior that sought to portray his bourgeois family's peculiar butler. The film is a reflection on the impossibility of such a project and the fact that he knew *a priori* what and how he intended to represent Santiago.

115 'Fossils Have a Hard Life: Apropos of the Image', *infra*, p. 138.

116 'What Is Not Seen (by the Self)', *infra*, p. 235.

117 See, for example, 'The Distinctiveness of the IMAGEs', *infra*, p. 181.

118 One can think of course of critiques of the overburdening of culture and memory, such as those developed, for instance, in *On the Genealogy of Morality*. In an unpublished text entitled *Être sans avoir* (*Being Without Having*) stored at the IMEC archives, likely contemporary to 'The Distinctiveness of the IMAGEs', Deligny does indeed mention Nietzsche. His critique of culture and civilisation is no doubt also related to his readings of authors such as Jean-Jacques Rousseau and Lévi-Strauss, who emphasised the notion that there is no progress without damage—*pas davantage sans dommage*: 'But "like us" implies a necessary belief in the validity of this "us," of the-humans-that-we-are [*le bonhomme*, the "everyman"] as we think and conceive of ourselves, after millennia of symbolic domestication, and Lord knows what advantages humanity has drawn from this. But at the expense of what? – this is what we still have to find out. There is no advantage without damage' ('The missing voice', in *The Arachnean and Other Texts, op. cit.*, p. 206). All these problems are synthetised in the motif of the 'detriment' that appears in the 'The Distinctiveness of the IMAGEs' (see *infra*, p. 186): 'Since language has existed—and all that it allows: the detriment.'

119 The motif of the 'asylum' appears in a number of texts contemporary to 'The Distinctiveness of the IMAGEs'. Indeed, Deligny gives it the positive sense of refuge, protection, shelter, and throughout his work, he describes the network for autistic children as a sort of asylum for another form of life. His reflection on the asylum is of particular interest today. We might also consider Donna Haraway's emphasis on a similar preoccupation when thinking about the need for refuge: 'Perhaps the outrage meriting a name like Anthropocene is about the destruction of places and times of refuge for people and other critters. [...] The Anthropocene marks severe discontinuities; what comes after will not be like what came before. I think our job is to make the Anthropocene as short/thin as possible and to cultivate with each other in every way imaginable epochs to come that can replenish refuge. Right now, the earth is full of refugees, human and not, without refuge' ('Anthropocene, Capitalocene, Plantationocene, Chthulucene: Making Kin', in *Environmental Humanities*, vol. 6, No. 1, pp. 159–165, p. 160, https://doi.org/10.1215/22011919-3615934).

120 'The Distinctiveness of the IMAGEs', *infra*, p. 214 and p. 222.
121 'Singulière Ethnie, ou l'Être et l'être', end of 1979, unpublished, in IMEC Archives.
122 'The Distinctiveness of the IMAGEs', *infra*, p. 173. It is indeed, as Silvia Rivera Cusicanqui puts it, a sort of 'logic of the included third', of the 'ch'ixi' ('Ch'ixinakax utxiwa: A Reflection on the Practices and Discourses of Decolonization', in *South Atlantic Quarterly*, vol. 111, No. 1, 2012, pp. 95–109, p. 105, https://doi.org/10.1215/00382876-1472612). Cusicanqui thinks, with this term, of a 'contradictory equilibrium that is even interwoven with irreducible differences' (Silvia Rivera Cusicanqui, *Un mundo ch'ixi es posible. Ensayo desde un presente en crisis*, Buenos Aires, Tinta Limón, 2018, p. 56, my translation).

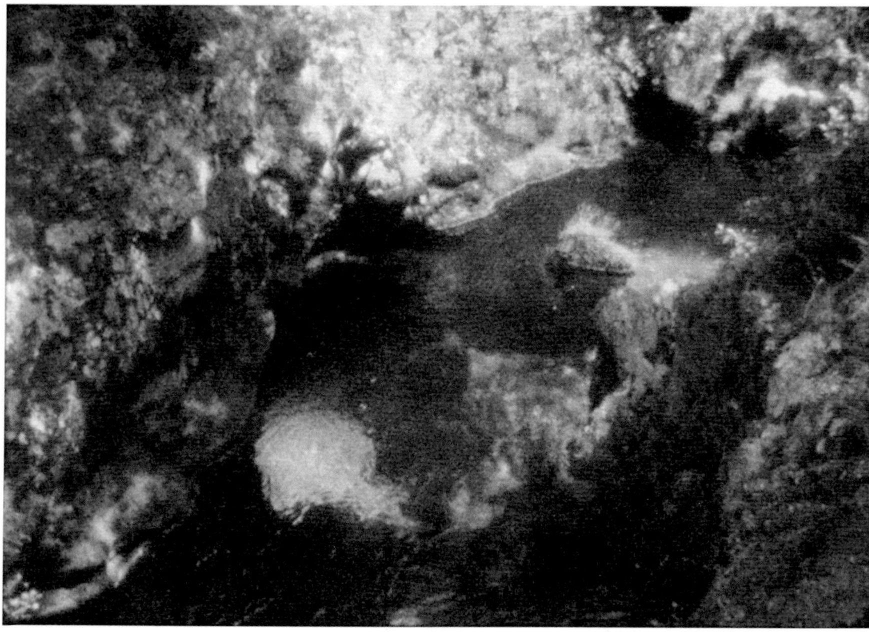

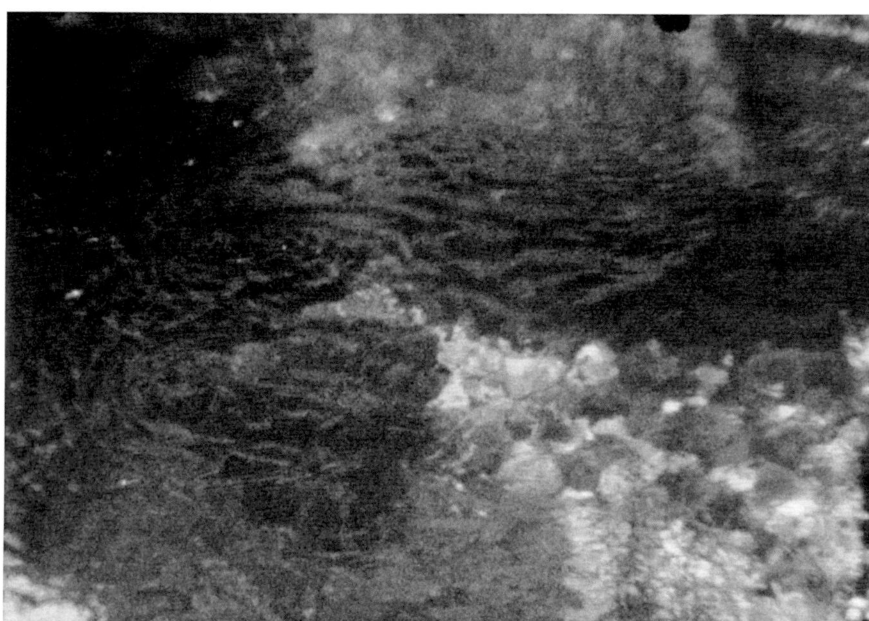

Shots of a river taken with a super 8 camera by Jacques Lin or Rose-Marie Ursenbach, 1984-1985.

Cinema. Cine-Club [1934][1]

Pierre HIRSCH is at it once again. On the 29th, he presented us with a careful selection of 'avant-garde' films.[2] Man Ray's *L'Étoile de mer* (*The Starfish*): images pass without logical connection, without 'history'.[3] In it, cinema is no longer photography. There is something else (perhaps only a frosted glass) that makes this short film into a moving painting with stock tricks; a masterpiece. Each gesture borrows symbolic value from the vaudeville ditty. Man Ray seeks: some people laugh and yet their ears hear a melody and they don't try to understand; they enjoy themselves. Why don't their eyes enjoy the melodies?

Ruttmann set images to Schumann's music.[4] And since Schumann had composed his piece with simple notes, Ruttmann composed his film with simple elements, with water, wind; he shows us lakes and boats, and the evening, and leaves rattling, and waterfalls and streams; the splashing of water after an outpouring of notes. The audience understands and doesn't complain that dreams have been imposed on them; and yet?

The third film, *The Trunks of Mr. O.F.*, has been reviewed.[5] I no longer know what the critics said. To me, it's a full-length film about a simple idea. The beginning is perfect, and then the effects become heavy-handed—nothing fails, nothing is silly, it's just that Granowsky is rather logical in his fantasising. I missed *L'Étoile de mer.*

If you would like to see different films, if you would like to see the curious results obtained by those who seek to photograph or recreate nature, those who, tired of words, compose poems of images, help your mate Hirsch out.

Join the Cine-Club, because Paris is faraway, the Rue de Béthune is full of duds, and 'films' are expensive.

Notes

1 Deligny wrote 'Cinéma. Ciné-club' in December of 1934. It was published at this time in the 8th issue of *Lille Université*.

2 The screening took place in Lille on November 29, 1934.

3 Man Ray, director, *L'Étoile de mer*, 1928.

4 Walter Ruttmann, director, *In der nacht*, 1931.

5 Alexis Granowsky, director, *The Trunks of Mr. O.F.*, 1931.

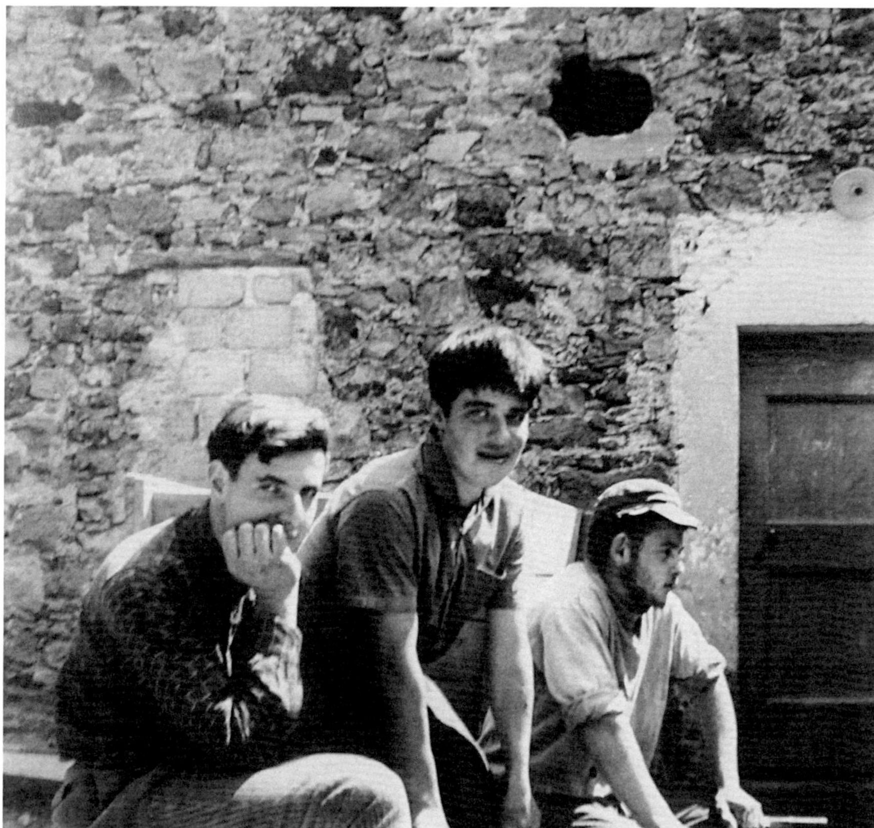

La Grande Cordée's participants (Yves Guignard, centre), around 1958.

The Camera, a Pedagogical Tool [1955][1]

The project of realising a documentary film that would be the collective work of the members of La Grande Cordée, regardless of their age, was born of the fact that cinema is a 'language' that is all the more important to us educators dealing with adolescents who, for the most part, hardly use written language—or don't at all—for lack of sufficient education, and whose spoken language is limited, not in terms of abundance, but in terms of the exchange value of the words and sentences used. They're talkative for the sake of talking, and language stupefies or fails them when it comes to making themselves understood.

They thus don't belong to a special category: over the course of their fifteen or seventeen years of existence, they have quite simply drained themselves of a rather cumbersome portion of the most common habits and customs of their time and milieu of life.

Images—photographs from newspapers and magazines, cinema, television—invade the world and deliver a permanent assault on written language. Spoken language doesn't elude the omnipresence of modern techniques of dissemination. I'll give just one example, that of Christian T., a brave and frail boy of fifteen, who becomes agitated and mute at the slightest question asked of him, and for whom elation is unleashed on hearing a word that allows him to recite a radio slogan. If he hears '*blanc*', he sings '*blancheur Persil*' or '*dents blanches, haleine fraîche*',[2] as happy as a duck in its pond to find himself once again on the commercial radio waves. As for the rest of the slogan, he has his own approach, his thoughts stumbling as he misses rhythms and words.

Let's leave Radio-Luxembourg behind and return to images. Magazine-photos, comic strips, cinema are just the facts. What would be the point of heroically defending the time of the first periodicals, when sentence and word, as specifically human, were queen and king and reigned supreme over title and text? It's likely that the image, the comic, the photo, are also specifically human, and so it's difficult to imagine people losing—little by little—use of the word, and thus thought, due to the abundance of images directly reproduced.

Cinema is thus an at-least weekly occurrence in the lives of the adolescents we need to help find a way out of an impasse that is only personal in appearance. To say that cinema as such does them wrong would be just as false as accusing literature of wrongdoing under the pretext of there being wrongful books.

Evidence . . . Evidence that one must take a closer look. From the moment a child sees a drawing, they draw, or at least are aware of the act of doing so. With theatre, the child immediately knows what it consists of: they speak and mime themself. Cinema, they endure. One watches a film a little as one watches a mountain or the sea. Even a street and houses are a reality the child or adolescent knows is authored, created by, people—their fellow beings, their elders: a child, whether a boy or girl, plays at making a house. But a film? Now film offers you 'reality' photographed. One doesn't feel a person has made a film as one does a drawing, for example.

I have never seen children play at making a film. It's true I have not seen every child play, but I believe they're 'ignorant' of the exact proportion of person in cinematographic creation, even if they know how a film is made. Film gives an initial impression of reality directly reproduced—a reality extracted from natural reality.

For me, there resides the force majeure and latent danger of cinema. The 'wings' of the cinematographic show are so faraway, so discrete, that a film is an event and no longer a show. It's not necessary for children to believe that what they see at the cinema is a raw sample of reality. What they need to know is that cinema entails a 'language'. They can only truly know this if they try the 'language' out themselves in order to perceive it without becoming spellbound by it. I thought that cinema would have a place in an organisation such as ours that seeks to help struggling adolescents. It's evidently not a question of each adolescent having their own camera, though it is necessary for the tool to truly be at the disposition of those who wish to use it in order to tell, in a few sequences of images, what they see of the life they live. As a teacher, I arranged for the dip pens (these were red and all alike: a painted wooden stick with the pen's metal nib, a lance-like nib, on the end; stirring; lagging behind the history of civilisation; eternal) to sit in full view on the desks, in their slots, even when the schoolchildren were not there, like the machinery at a construction site at dawn, before the workers arrive.

As an educator, I want to see the tool for capturing images ready to use—a complicated tool with its internal mechanism and turrets, but one that inspires a salutary respect in the most indifferent and careless of scoundrels.

How have we made use of it thus far?

Poorly, it goes without saying, and in a quite parsimonious manner, given the cost of film and its processing. But in the end, the camera is there, and to continue the comparison with writing, let's just say that some of La Grande Cordée's boys, as well as the adults who are part of the same organisation, did very little scribbling before arriving at sentences—that is, at sequences.

Three-quarters of the film that was shot is still lying around in some laboratory, the consequence, as always, of the much-talked-about money. It's thus not a matter of speaking of the 'oeuvre'—of the film—considering its current state. We have not yet seen the reels shot in the Vercors last July. There were a good fifteen or so of us camping right at the foot of the Deux-Soeurs. The camera moved from hand to hand, rattling away. At what scenario?

The scenario was vast, inordinately vast for the five or six thirty-metre reels that we had available. We were in the Vercors, one of the centres of the Resistance. There were seventeen of us: fifteen boys aged thirteen to eighteen who arrived at the Deux-Soeurs eight days before us adults. One of them, a sixteen-year-old, was in charge; a disturbed individual, he had as bad a reputation as the others. With them was a young woman aged twenty. They had a large white tent that would not remain tethered to the ground when the wind rasped the mountains. One night, they had to get up and tether it, tying the ropes amid gusts of rain. The next day, a peasant offered them a hut that had not sheltered anyone since the time of the Maquis.

The film was there, ready to be made. Fifteen boys looking everywhere for the Maquis: along the paths, in the memory of the people. Fifteen boys who would have asked, camera in hand, for the pieces of the Maquis's history to be relived; a mise en scène once again; played, after having been lived, by those two peasants, survivors of Pas-de-l'Aiguille; by that elderly man who spoke with enemy patrols while beneath the hay in his barn the 'terrorists' didn't dare breathe. That film was not made.

There were many other films projected that would not be realised either.

For example, along with the past members of La Grande Cordée, we would have liked to try and film what the fourteen- or sixteen-year-old boys see of the neighbourhood they're from; what they perceive in the labyrinth of streets around their house; in order for the camera to show what their eyes see of this familiar reality each day, and what these same eyes see a few months later—a few months having been spent elsewhere, far from home, among other people, grappling with another 'regimen for living', once some intention of a future occupation has been developed. To try and show how a set of new intentions modify the perception of reality.

Such is the document we attempted for a few months.

But events didn't allow us to linger on this pursuit.

A secondary camera would have been needed and we have just the one, automatically occupied so as to be the most useful—not for recording pedagogical activity, but for participating in this activity, a little like a lone, unique, and valued mechanical weapon in combat. What is the combat in question?

For the most part, the boys come to us lacking concrete intentions. At best, they come presenting words such as 'mason' or 'live independently . . . '—meagre passports for the future. Nevertheless, we leave our stamp in them: the words of hope we try to nourish in the transient population that is the small collectivity that makes up the orientation week.

The camera is at the disposition of the boy in charge of the week's scheduling.

Every night, after we meet for an hour, each of the boys in the orientation week writes down their schedule for the next day as precisely as possible.

The boy in charge of individual scheduling for the week checks if, at the time specified, each boy has done what he planned—what he selected the day prior for work, task, or leisure, among the regular or occasional options of work and tasks available: building construction, decorating projects, gardening, giving a hand to neighbouring farmers, maintenance and household work, trial apprenticeships with artisans nearby, and all that which a market town and village in the Haute-Loire can offer as activities of every kind.

If, over the course of his rounds, the boy in charge for the week perceives a 'scene' that he finds interesting, and he's capable of operating the camera, he films it. If not, he calls an 'operator'—that is, another boy who's already sufficiently experienced, so as not to waste the film.

It often happens that one of the past members of La Grande Cordée writes or comes to see where things stand with the new recruits, or that a boy who has left for a trial placement returns to the orientation week to refocus his intentions. The film, snippets of which were shot by all, is the object of the first remarks exchanged. How's the film coming? It's the organisation's memory, a memory struck by long periods of amnesia, though I believe that when we're able to carry out a first edit of the reels, we'll have something better than a collective memory: we'll have the beginnings of a consciousness unique to the collectivity of La Grande Cordée.

Makarenko insists on the force of custom in a pedagogical collectivity.

Our attempt, a dispositive of trial placements that spread La Grande Cordée's boys out towards the conditions of existence assumed to be favourable to their development, doesn't lend itself well to the establishment of customs and traditions that, via attitudes, transmit the collective experience from individual to individual.

Our pedagogical collectivity, in its fight against enemy forces (that is: the lack of apprenticeship, the 'morals' of the decaying classes, in which contradictions and philosophies find favourable ground in the weakest of mentalities, even in the form of slang expressions) should draw inspiration from a more maquisard 'strategy'.

The hundred or so kids in the Gorki community were able to form a united front in a society in the process of organising its future prospects.

For our kids, forming a united front would be forming a target. They multiply their chances of getting by when they spread out in a country where nothing but their exploitation as unstable labourers is conscientiously planned.

And yet they're in need of a 'collectivity'—or, if one wishes, a supportive milieu—that informs them of, and 'inspires' in them, a somewhat consistent and sustained means of acquiring raisons d'être, because for the most part, they feel themselves to be in the way on an earth where it seems everything takes place as though they had nothing to do there. The film gives them a raison d'être. They have something to prove. They have been treated as individuals who are disturbed, retarded, 'sick', a waste of space. They could become role models. With the camera, the world looks at them, the world of the Others who had nothing to do with them, and who will later be the witnesses to what they do every day.

Mise en scène? No. *Mise en vue. Mise au clair. Mise en public.* Placed in view. Put straight. Made public.

While I write, the camera is on my table, without ammunition. We have no film left again, after two days. The automatic weapon is mute. Beyond my head, on the slabs of the orientation week's long corridor, which is conducive to the chase, the infantry goes to great lengths to clean the dust that the feudal building where we live perspires in all its nooks and crannies. It's 14 July 1955.

If all goes to my liking, they'll soon be fishing with a permit for five and a rod. Maurice A., who's seventeen years old, has said he won't go. For him, the enemy is the pub. The enemy is numerous. Maurice A. hides. He was filmed grappling with plaster and cement on the small construction site he started when he arrived. He knows that if he starts drinking again, the piece of film in which he exists as foreman of the construction site will be put aside for a long time, until he truly lives a life in harmony with the first images.

And if it's true, as I believe it is, that new intentions modify what a being perceives of the world surrounding them, then Maurice A.—his cooperative future now in mind—is no longer on the same earth as Maurice A., the precocious drudge of a construction worker taught to drink by the companions who didn't want to do wrong, treating him as an equal when they passed the bottle they were drinking from themselves.

Vast world. The force of habits, trends, customs. In the face of them, it would be very imprudent to wish to immediately spark new intentions with the small and big words that have arisen after too many years of use by the hypocrisy of bourgeoisie morale. But what about with images?

La Grande Cordée, Salzuit near Paulhaguet (Haute-Loire)

Notes

1 'La caméra outil pédagogique' was written in 1955 and first published in the 97th issue of *Vers l'éducation nouvelle* in October-November of the same year.

2 If Christian T. hears the word *blanc*, 'white', he sings '*blancheur Persil*', 'Persil whiteness', from the Persil laundry detergent ad, or '*dents blanches, haleine fraîche*', 'white teeth, fresh breath', the Colgate toothpaste slogan at the time.

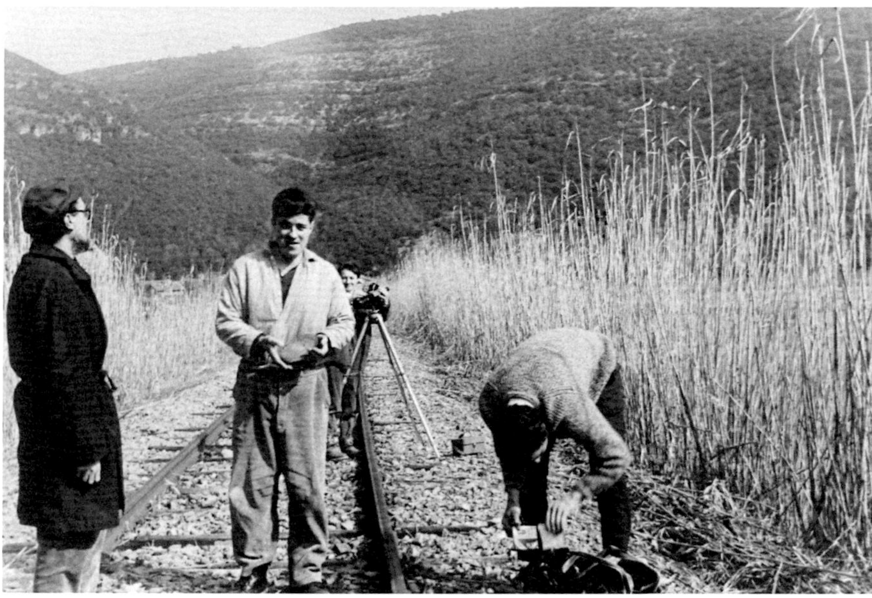

Image from the shooting of *The Slightest Gesture*.

He's Still One of Us [1971][1]

The film, *Le Moindre geste* (*The Slightest Gesture*), which I'm told 'was chosen by the Semaine de la Critique's selection committee and will thus be shown at Cannes', came very close to remaining rolled up in large tin cans that might have contained preserves, as so often happens to those 'abnormal' children for whom fate is rolled up in the places intended for them. And what can be done about this?

The fate common to the being I'm going to talk about and the kilometres of film that carry his image will perhaps clarify a little what I mean when I talk about attempt.

A film can be a masterpiece or a dud; a small celebration or an adhesive strip that captures ideas in the spirit of the times like sticky paper did flies, back when it was used and bicycles filled the streets.

That Yves, who's 'severely retarded', escaped his fate, which was to live in a home for halfwits—*demeurer dans une demeure à demeurés*—and that this strange film did not remain eternally autistic—as is the case with abandoned objects—entail two events that merge into one.

Yves and his father *étaient là*—they were here—earlier. The father spoke to me. Yves had picked up a pencil sharpener on my desk and was handling it with three fingers and that air of his that involves seeing a lot more in an object than its common use—of which he's suspicious. In 1957, *ils étaient là*, but at the time, *là* was there, in the Allier, and his father had said to me that we ought to destroy the wall he saw, an adobe wall four or five metres high that was the surviving part of a destroyed barn. Yves didn't say anything, caught up as he was in the habit of never addressing his speech to anyone; he was clumsy, ruddy, black-haired, bumbling, and placed a wall of silence between 'the rest of us' and himself; and though there could not have been any more human there, nor more of all that which life entails, it took us years, walking side by side, day after day, and from place to place, from the Allier to the Cévennes, to make the film that 'would thus be shown at Cannes'.

I very much fear the damn wall that echoes what everyone says back to them, that it will rise up again, between the screen and those who watch the filmed document, which could have been titled *Le royaume des cieux* (*The Kingdom of Heaven*)—except that this title was the property of an academician. I chose: *The Slightest Gesture*; the clandestine subtitle: *What are its roots?*

My project, which guided the shots taken, was to give those who would see the images their part of the being who I saw and heard living with us for six or seven years, just as he was in his attitudes, gestures, and remarks—familiar and haughty; his speech vacant then suddenly loquacious and vituperative, and in that spoken flood,

I recognised the speech that makes us what we are—so similar was it to Yves's—and that reigns, universal, historical, demonstrative, zany, deadly.

We set out: five of us, plus the camera, plus the other kid—a thirteen-year-old collected in the nearest town. The Cévennes are vast and the theme was clear: two adolescents escape from a psychiatric hospital, one who sprints in front and for whom running away comes as naturally as breathing, and the other, who follows him, and is mentally retarded and a little crazy, perhaps as a result of having lived among those who are.

I had said to Yves: 'It's you . . . in the film, it's you . . . but you would have spent four or five years living with people who are crazy . . . now you're free to go. . . .' The camera pointing at him, Yves began to impersonate Fernandel. The camera didn't shoot while that shade from the television passed, just as it didn't shoot when the clouds came and spoilt the light that was usually so generous we were able to shoot without a photocell, ignorant as we were of how to use this contraption that seemed to us so highly specialised.

After Fernandel, we were treated to a grand impression of de Gaulle, at which point shooting could begin, each site and what was encountered in it bringing about what happened in it. There was hardly any preliminary confabulation. It can't be said that Yves and the other kid were playing. They were struggling; they were in the film and in the sun, sometimes for hours, and it was July. What happened was that Yves began to bellow so loudly that the police, who had been alerted, arrived with an ambulance they had to leave on the road. They went from terrace to terrace and found us by the sound of his voice. All around us, in a long chain, in a vast casting net, such as children might form in a school courtyard, were the inhabitants, encircling us in a hunt straight out of the Middle Ages. We were there—the five of us, plus the other kid, plus the unpointing camera—in that house with the large roof open to the Cévennes sky that had in fact seen it all.

During periods of respite—in the evening, at night, at daybreak—Yves recorded that ruminating speech of his; he jabbered to his heart's content and filled the tapes of the cassette recorder he respected, slapping the grassy ground while he vociferated about the froth on his lips; froth that was drying, a tenacious fringe of speech, like the trace of the last tide one sees on the beach.

The following day, as soon as the light showed itself to be good, we set out again to discover, near Saint-Jean-du-Gard or close to Anduze, a site that would lend itself to Yves getting his bearings.

During this almost daily game, we took more than twenty hours of images without knowing what was on the film.

As to the film-monster, it's no surprise it remained locked up for years.

The person who said to me, 'I've got to edit that . . . ', must not have realised. I think he put two years into it, editing at night, as he had other things to do. . . . What remains is an hour and forty-five minutes of a film wed to what could be retained of the discourse that was so fascinating—an echo of all that is said, including at Mass—that Yves, on hearing himself think, allows his hands to become unclasped and to return, on their own, to the gestures of infancy. One need not be particularly clever to tell me whether here was a child or the being I continue, despite everything, to call human, even though his speech is not of this world.

At the start of this text, I wrote that the film is an attempt. Let me explain.

I saw the film edited, mixed . . . and in it, I found hardly any of my intentions—which could get jumbled up during shooting, and which continued to proliferate throughout the film's lengthy premature lock-up. However, certain scenes did seem to have been filmed only yesterday, taken from the 'position' I defend today, in the 'guerrilla' pursuit I undertake as best I can.

I often feel the same way about this strange 'oeuvre' that consists in attempting to get a child-fool out of trouble. If the child is forgotten, something comes of it. In sum, this is what happened to the film. The great lottery of circumstance. SLON took the baton in order for *The Slightest Gesture* to be released, while another attempt took the baton from the first, the film serving as both its tool and trace.[2]

The last time I saw the film before it left to be seen, Yves and almost all those who had been his companions during shooting were there, in a house in Monoblet. Yves said: 'Do you like it?'

This 'you' was directed towards those who would see who Yves is in the film.

Yves is burly, ruddy, always a little 'simple'; and yet, he's one of us. Sometimes he has to work and he goes about it like a horse. He *is* one of us, but one should not be misled, as he's not quite; still, he gets by—*il s'en tire*—now, without the person who persists in undertaking this attempt after the first, always in a group of five so things don't get out of hand, even if one individual replaces another. *Yves s'en tire.* As to the film, *lui, il est tiré*: it's ready. All that remains is to watch it.

If we had a camera and film, we would begin shooting again, the character no longer a being in person—a 'particular' one—but US, not the five of us, but US the rest of us, everybody and anybody, grappling with:

– How to *be human* around the severely psychotic children who come stay with us in the very Cévennes that provide a good excuse—these eroded remains of the Hercynian belt which, I'm told, was penetrated by the waters of the Flood itself.

On the flanks of the mountains reigns the evergreen oak that invades the terraces where the olive tree no longer grows. I find the light to be pristine, just as it was seven years prior when on seeing it we said: 'Let's go. . . .'

And we set out towards that quarry, the racket evoking, from afar, a fishing boat with a diesel engine on its last legs, taking forever to start. We were there along the

Gardon: five plus one—the kid who would remain in the hole, because for Yves, speech serves not for saying things but for making proclamations.

The children who live among us now are neither deaf nor mute. The majority have never said a word in their lives.

And what about US?

Notes

1 'Quand même il est des nôtres' was written in 1971 and first published in the 55th issue of *Jeune Cinéma* in May of the same year.

2 SLON, Société pour le lancement des œuvres nouvelles (Society for Launching New Works', later called ISKRA), was a cooperative formed by Chris Marker, among others, that produced and distributed films.

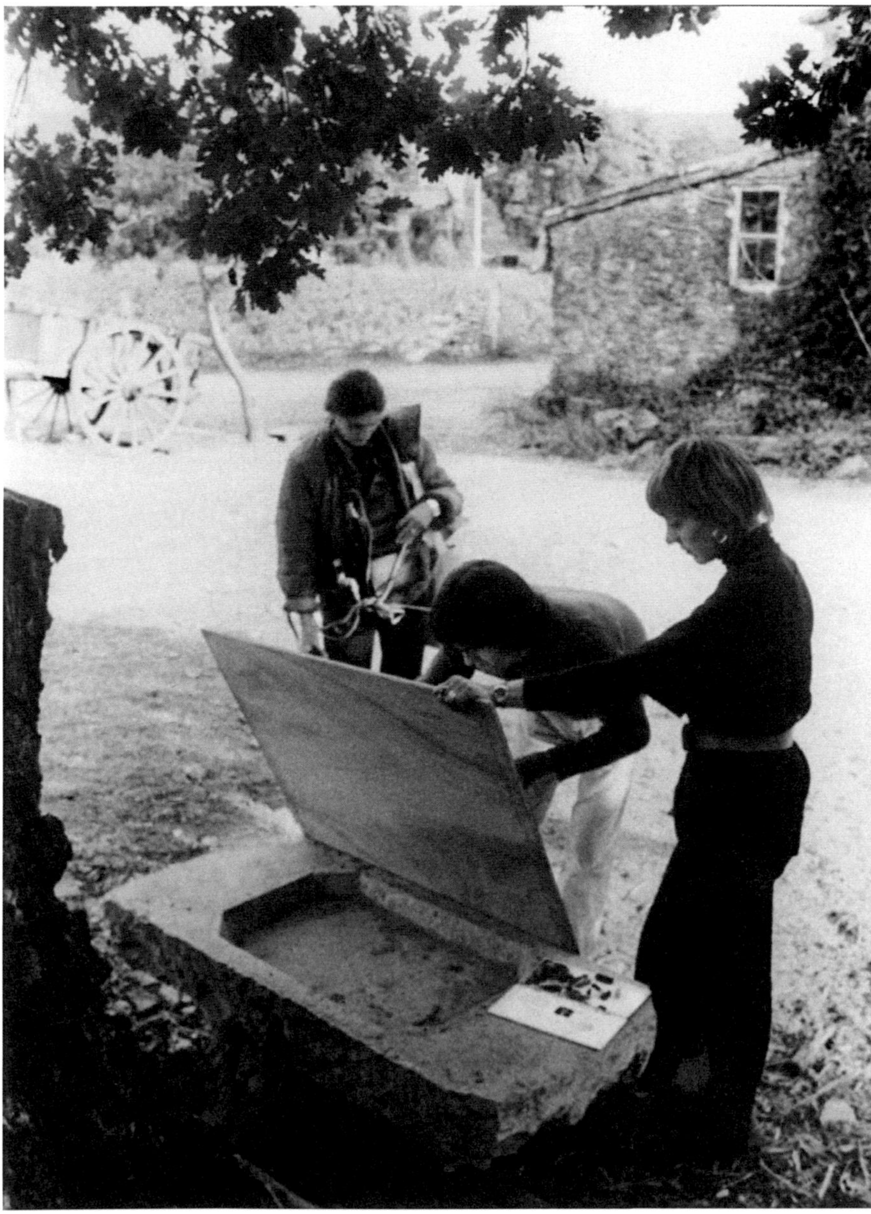

Caroline Deligny with the Paluche Camera, 1978-1979.

Camering [1977][1]

'Tools always presuppose a machine, and the machine is always social before being technical. There is always a social machine which selects or assigns the technical elements used.'

Gilles Deleuze[2]

One can think of the camera as a tool, an instrument, a machine that enables images to be recorded. These images can then be projected.

Words have a history. What the dictionary told us—in times past—of *projeter*, to project, was '*jeter dehors*', the image evoked being that of rejecting something, throwing it out, while the word *projet*, a project, which has the same origin, evokes 'all that by which people tend to modify the world or themselves in a given way'.

One is well aware that what's rejected is not worth much, is detritus. It's not particularly surprising that so many projections do indeed cause one to think of a rubbish dump on the outskirts of a village. Society takes out its rubbish and contemplates, and is moved by, the result of its effort. Society sees *itself* in the household rubbish that is projected in various formats. But what then is the Itself in question? Do people see themselves as they are? They see the leftovers, the packaging, the rejections, and are prompted to contemplate what they don't want, or no longer want, from their own customary. Nothing is lost. Projections are consumer goods. Thus functions a recovery circuit in which household rubbish holds on tight to what's imagined, projected.

One sees the S' functioning as a dominant instrument on a detour by way of the camera, that small chamber ruled, reigned over, by a *camérier*, or chamberlain, 'an officer in the pope or cardinal's chambers', or by a *camériste*, or chambermaid, 'a woman who attended to a princess'. On occasion, it's the *camerlingue*, or camerlengo: 'a cardinal of the papal court who administers justice and the treasury, presides over the apostolic chamber, and governs when the Holy See is vacant.'

This is the case in the *Petit Robert* dictionary, which makes no mention of the cameraman. Though it is true that he who shoots a film occasionally takes himself to be the pope.

What about a *scénario*, a screenplay? The word comes from '*cène*', the Last Supper. Which is a surprise. Either the proofreader of the *Petit Robert* wasn't on the ball or what we're now dealing with is the Eucharist, and an author who's thus sharing his *manière de voir*, his way of seeing, with us. Now, from *voir* to *voirie,*[3] a refuse dump, all that's missing is a syllable, the referred-to rubbish evoked once again.

Since I spoke of a detour by way of the camera, it would seem as though the camera were a *place*, which is altogether different from just being the box that projects the camerlengo's mischievous ways, the camerlengo not being the least concerned with modifying the world or himself in any which way; camerlengo or chambermaid, the prince will be well-served, whether he's the pope or a tyrant or simply power.

So it is that one must keep an eye on what could take place in, and by virtue of, that small chamber that is entirely black on the inside, even invent the infinitive of a verb that could be 'to camer', which would entail all that 'to camerleng' or 'to chambermaid' would not.

Let's imagine someone who's somewhat tormented by the desire to write, which is common enough—each of us is capable of experiencing the urge to express ourself and has the right to do so. Those who manage to publish a book seem privileged. Among individuals who wish to obtain this privilege, there are those who feel themselves to be disabled, handicapped, either with regard to spelling, or grammar: the instrument is lacking, while the camera reassures them with its built-in mechanism, thanks to which the film is made by itself, so to speak. It's a godsend. The camera used as a prosthesis for wobbly writing is a very common occurrence.

The happenstances of existence have resulted in the opposite fate in my case. Equipped with writings that have been published and are read to some degree, it was the making of a film that I was missing. It seemed to me that if I had been able to save images of what had taken place here or there, in the frame of what could be seen, the rawest of images, they would have sounded, all on their own, like bells, nothing but these images. And the advantage, which seemed to me enormous, was that these raw images didn't carry with them a single belief. It's there that the camerlengo disappears.

I'll give a brief example: in Lille, where I lived at the time, there were ramparts that remained intact after Vauban. And atop those ramparts was the municipal refuse dump, which then made use of horse-drawn wagons that transported and unloaded the abundant waste produced and left out each day in the bins lined up along the city's sidewalks. This disposed waste formed a heap. A support horse awaited the arrival of each wagon; harnessed in front of the other horse, which, on flat land, was up to the task, the support horse helped pull the wagon to the top of the heap. The cart was tipped and its contents tumbled down the slopes in cascades. Now, on the slopes stood elderly residents from the nursing home and neighbourhood children. Among them, a young girl with long hair who must have been four or five years old. She was watching the avalanches.

I took to making a customary detour of that place. One day, during the course of an avalanche, there tumbled down a lamp fixture the likes of which one doesn't see any more. It's true that one hardly ever sees an empress's crown nowadays. But that gas lamp fixture, perched on the girl's head, her whole body holding it in balance there, was just that: an extravagant, splendid crown. The elderly men and women from the nursing home had settled in on the mountainside, each with a hand propped on the ground to form a tripod, watching. On the horizon, and in the frame, were the columns of the Palais de Justice, and a bit farther behind them, the very high walls of the prison and their barred windows. This gave them the appearance of being made up, with very heavy eyelashes.

You might tell me that such occurrences are rare. Perhaps. That is why one must go about camering.

One must read what Deleuze says about stirrups being one with the times.[4]

The camera might be something not unlike those stirrups, thanks to which our gaze is supported, each of us taking off, astride a horse, eyes half-closed . . . astride what? The camerlengo hastens to provide the horse, put otherwise, the letter of credit; the chambermaid shines its hooves, even though the stirrups would be sufficient.

That such an occurrence is rare—the prison, the Palais de Justice, the piling up of household rubbish on the fringe of the city, elderly men and women in uniform, horses, empress girl—is true.

The images that were concentrated in the frame—all that had to be done was centre them—could have been scattered throughout the city and its periphery. For the camera to take these scattered images and, by virtue of the mystery of that small black chamber, go about making them neighbours, attracted within the frame as filings by a magnet, that magnet can't be the SELF of-someone-who-tells-themself-something-in-order-that-others-tell-themselves-what-they-tell-themself-and-want-others-to-believe. Nothing new here: it's a question of *montrer*, of showing, so to speak, where the horse can be found. And the *monture*, the mount, in question? Isn't the *monteur*, the film editor, just a *montreur*, a showperson?

Imagine the images I have evoked in writing: childhood and old age, the nursing home and justice, the outdoors and what's indoors, the horses, the avalanche, the serfs and the moujiks, and the sky and hell, because the former smoked at the level of the slopes—the rubbish heap that slowly consumed itself a volcano at rest.

Who would dare interfere, and in one way or another, stick their nose into a scene that one sees is not about painting, or music, or writing? Must one take people for fools to so great an extent as to imagine what they should see for them, or worse, tell them what that is? I would say that the telling of it is worse because mishandled images, strung together in a certain, advised way, still allow one to see something other than that which the street performer intends to show or demonstrate—*montrer* or *démontrer*.

One might say to me: 'But this is no more than a moment. It does not a film make.'

Better perhaps an instant made film than so many films without an ounce of 'instant'. I'm talking about camering and not screenplaying. Numerous enough are those who carry out the latter.

But what I can do is disengage myself from that instant in order to describe another aspect that can be evoked by camering—and this without leaving the path I'm on.

There were seven of us: five behind and two in front, in the frame. None of us had the least experience handling that contraption we call a camera. That said, what we did have was time—the months, the years—so to speak, in the frame. One might tell me that time is not filmed. But when it comes to the camera, *le temps*, meaning both time and the weather, matters. In addition to the latter, on which the light depends, there is the time that passes. The images that had been taken and rolled up, a copy of the work stored in flat cans of preserves, remained there, intact, two years later—an autistic-like memory where all that has been seen can reappear at any instant, which is to say that every instant filmed can reverberate with the echoes of other instants whose images surface after they have passed.

That memory, for our purposes, really took *place* in those tin cans, an archive of sorts, out of which came the subject and title of a film that was not at all pre-viewed: *Le Moindre geste* (*The Slightest Gesture*). Here it can be seen how a project that has a certain objective can, at any point, be diverted, its intent suddenly drying up.

An example: the two individuals, the film's characters, were escaping from a mental asylum, one following the other, as it goes, and it so happened that the other inadvertently found himself in a pit, a cellar he would clearly be unable to climb out of if not for the involvement of the one following. And the one in question, who was asyled to the core, having spent more than ten years of his life in the hospital he only ever left to follow the other, not *for* any reason, but as if there were no possible reason, wanders about in the vicinity of the pit from which the other's cries are coming. He wanders somewhat idly and, not looking for anything in particular, finds a pickaxe. So he goes about wielding the pickaxe with force and violence beyond what's called for. And the pickaxe's handle breaks in two. The iron loses its handle. There thus remain two pieces of wood. With a bit of wire twisted around them by the hero and supposed rescuer, the pieces of wood obstinately form a cross. And upon realising that it's now a cross he has in his hands, it occurs to him to hold a procession all on his own with the aim of proceeding, as is the custom, to a burial, during which the right thing to do is mutter prayers. The other's cries become an entirely inopportune occurrence, superfluous, as it were, bird cries like those heard in nature while we're bustling about.

Here it's evident that all of us are buried in advance by what could be referred to as the predominance of a certain order, which though symbolic is no less dominant, and that the cross of belief[5] is ideology itself, religious or otherwise.

As for the find that emerged in these images, I hope you'll take my word for it when I say it was not preconceived. I'll reiterate: we had the time, the hero's gestures followed their course like weeds sprouting up. One needs time to film weeds sprouting up. The roll of film came very close to remaining in the tin cans *in aeternam* for several reasons: we had run out of money; none of us was, to a greater or lesser extent, professionally involved in the cinematic institution; I had no story to show, to champion and promote.

No one believed the fact that there could be a film in those tin cans. Ten years of common existence for some, three of which were spent camering: ten hours of images rolled up in two or three flat tin cans meant that no one could question it—what was in there was a film, edited, as chance would have it, by someone from elsewhere. And that film was selected for the parallel section of the Festival de Cannes in I can no longer recall which year.

I'll say no more so as to encourage those who would not otherwise venture to undertake *camering*.

I would additionally say to them that what *camering* entails is a long-term undertaking and that it's thus a question of the attempt; it's not at all necessary to see the end since if you could, you would fear not having the means to get there.

I maintain that *camering* doesn't come to an end, and it's perhaps here that it differs from filming, or as it's commonly put, realising a film, just as one would say writing a novel. But then it's the book that is written or the film that is made. Not that I disdain those works that *do* have to be made.

Camering is a question of something else, which could be written as camerring,[6] as though a certain *point de voir*, a point of seeing, were to wander in an attempt. Would this attempt be that of making a film? Not at all. An attempt takes place(s), with the camera incorporated, so to speak, in the customary. Was the film thus not staged? It was not. We're not at the theatre.

There is a certain *point of seeing* that retains traces of what takes place in the frame that is distinct to it.

Afterwards, one must of course edit, a task for which one doesn't necessarily require large horses stomping about with the ideas they see coming—from a distance. One recognises them: they're always the same.

While the hero of the 'slightest gesture' returned from the river with cans of preserves full of water so that the other, in his pit, could drink—the other having shouted at him plenty: 'A drink . . . go to the river'—he happened upon a house en route, an empty, abandoned house, among the others, which were deserted as well. He sat down on the doorstep. On the ceiling, the sun's light reflected off the water in one of the cans. The hero gathered up the cans to make his way towards the other, because the other was not there. Can removed, reflection gone. Now the reflection was missing from the cracked ceiling of that empty dwelling, and its absence was a serious matter. So the hero placed the cans back in the sun, on the doorstep. On the ceiling, the reflection danced gaily.

You might say to me: 'What of it? That doesn't mean a thing. . . .' It's thus *camering*, distinctly speaking.

Notes

1 Written in 1978, the first 'Camérer' piece to appear in this volume was originally published in the 53rd issue of *Trafic* in the spring of 2005. It was called 'Camérer #2' in *Camérer. À propos d'images*, Paris, L'Arachnéen, 2021.

2 Gilles Deleuze and Claire Parnet, *Dialogues*, translated by Hugh Tonlinson and Barbara Habberjam, New York, Columbia University Press, 1987, p. 70.

3 The word *voirie* is more commonly used to refer to a public road network or the department responsible for such.

4 *Ibid.*, p. 72.

5 Here Deligny plays with the paronyms *croix* and *croire*, 'cross' and 'belief', respectively.

6 In French, Deligny suggests the neologism *camerrer*, which contains the verb *errer*, 'to wander'.

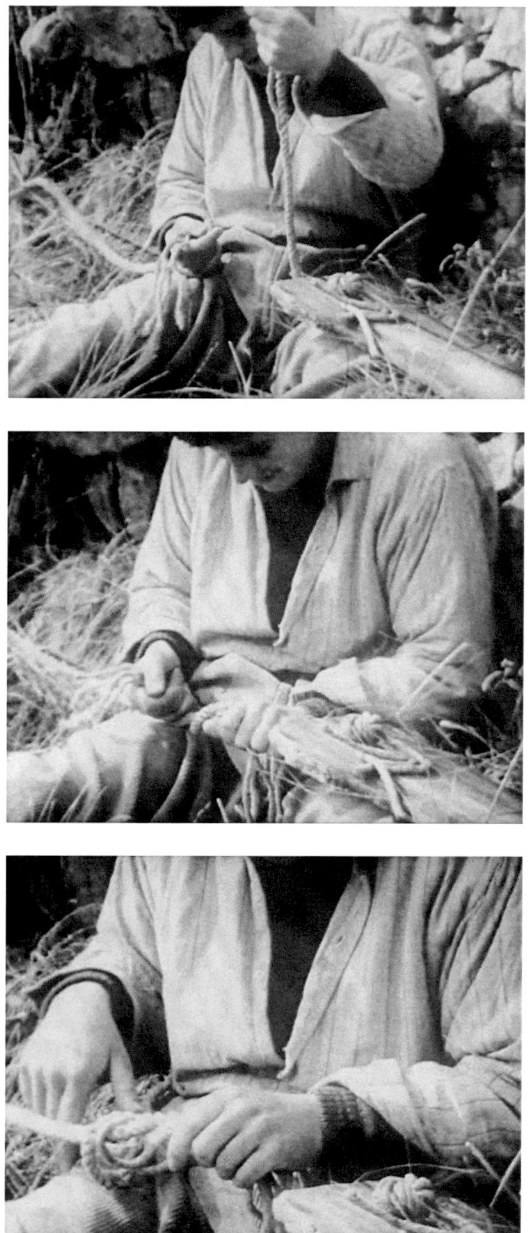

Photograms from *The Slightest Gesture*.

Miscreating [1979][1, 2]

To discuss the infinitive that is the banner over this work[3]

A belief in god has always—and now more than ever—seemed the convention. It may be a better alloy than a belief in people for those who believe themselves to be non-believers. As for people who do believe, they're the direct heir of those who came to be in times past, when a belief in god was unanimous, or nearly so.

For people who don't believe—in the supernatural—it's a matter of not taking over, in good faith, from the person who projects themself, who's immutable, or nearly so. But it's to be expected that this rupture is just barely repaired, endlessly—people holding on to their image just as they did that of god. It's the same thing.

The space of an attempt is, for me, the space of a rupture. It's not that I myself need to break away from some belief, having never inherited a belief—in the supernatural. Instead, it's a matter of breaking away from the image acquired of the person, of myself, of others—but rather than acquired, incorporated: I want to talk about the inveterate image in which the thousand and one ways people have regarded themselves, and regard themselves, are focused, reiterated, and condensed; the 'self' supplanting, substituting, the human that everyone, in good conscience, can't help but be unaware of, people's consciousness eclipsing, in good faith, the human that is not its responsibility, and which it must expel in order to further its influence.

Put otherwise, consciousness is totalitarian, and the human always/already liminal.

MisCreating, which is the banner over the connected texts gathered here, doesn't evoke a different way for people to imagine themselves. The beliefs derived from believing are varied; they may appear disparate and contradictory; they may boast of materialist good sense. They inevitably share a point of coherence, an inevitable focal point; put otherwise, they share the *one* in every that is to the human what a reflection on the ceiling or beneath the arch of a bridge is to the water that does the reflecting. To take the reflection for the water is to take the person for the human. But while water doesn't suffer as a result of this mistake, the human is eliminated.

Hence it being necessary to misCREATE, even if it's only the space of an attempt, which necessitates the implementation of a practice that has proven necessary in our daily lives after twelve years of living close to autistic children. The further we went, the more steps forward we took in our approach, and the more it became clear that we were looking for an art of living that would allow these children to exist.

It may be that all the arts have something in common, just as the sciences do.
Hence the idea, the project, of carrying out another attempt, all while respecting the space-time of the first, which entails a practice based on the work of *tracing*, of retaining traces. All that was needed was a change of instruments. This other attempt would be given the infinitive *to camer*, a different way of retaining traces. It would involve images-sounds taken, and no longer linear traces transcribed.

Just as it occurred to me to chronicle the first approach, I'll now describe the space-time and practice we seek. Just as tracing is not drawing, *camering* is not filming.

To Fulfil or to Disappoint?

While we're here, discussing art, what I think is that it's a question of disappointing rather than fulfilling. Those who have on occasion created—as is said of the artist—have deliberately, and this was no doubt stronger than them, evaded fulfilling the wishes and desires of their contemporaries. They discovered another function, another role, than that of satisfying others.

It's not easy to disappoint; every work creates a mirage, each of us mirrored in it. For the creator, the need for approval seems to be taken to a bit of an extreme; this is often true, though not at all when it's a matter of an attempt, that is, of a breach whereby the human—that people are not at all conscious of—takes *forms*.

Which is to state the importance of *forms* that are recognised as entailing something other than the sharing of intentions or convictions.

Intentions and Convictions

Does this mean that the everyone we are at the start of this other attempt has neither intentions nor convictions? That would be to claim we don't have consciousness of being. We do have them—of that there is no doubt. Our project is neither to share them nor to convince. We don't have an idea of the person, a truth to disseminate. There is reality as it's felt, which just so happens to be rather unanimous, whether or not this appears to be the case, and there is the real. If the real is that which eludes language, certain aspects of it might appear in images.

The camera is an instrument that exists and whose use is widespread. There must be some other way to handle this instrument that evades what it's usually tasked with doing;[4] a way that attempts to break the tacit pact between the person who films and the one who watches the film.

To break this pact is to risk disappointing others.

I happened to make—so to speak—a film. The hero was so severely retarded that he couldn't tie a knot with two ends of rope. Meanwhile, the other character, his companion, was dying of thirst and fear in a pit he was unable to climb out of on his own.

Without suspecting as much, I was already inclined *to camer* rather than to film.

As for the other character, in the pit, nothing could be seen of him. It was quite dark at the bottom of that pit, and we didn't have the means—the money necessary—to illuminate it in such a way as is possible with filming. Meanwhile, the hero wasn't able to tie the knot, this taking place in full sunlight: him, his hands and his head, and the rest, and the two ends of rope.

The images in this film—there were a good ten hours of them—were abandoned in their large tin can, as I was caught up in, seized by, that other attempt that was living close to autistic children. And the images happened to move on to editing, which implied a *monteur*, or editor, who, working two hundred kilometres from where I was, realised, so to speak, what he could with those images, in the space-time allotted to the projection of a film—a hundred minutes or so. I continued to feel remorse for having abandoned what seemed to me the real find: two hands that aren't able to tie a knot, that go on not being able for an eternity. In the hundred minutes or so that was the length given to the projected film, what should have been shown—for at least half the allotted time, or a little more than half for good measure—were those hands that weren't able; that was where the drama was. Because after all, why should one care who kills who in a film, or who doesn't love whoever loves them, or about any of the other things one has seen so many times that by now they hold no interest. Whereas the two hands of a human being that aren't able to tie a knot—now that's surprising. It's true there is the other kid, who's on the verge of death not far away, and that what's happening is the knot that isn't tied. What should have been seen were those two hands at work, unrelenting and ineffective. Some viewers might have thought: 'He's got to hurry up with that knot; he's got to help the other kid out.' And they would have been mistaken, since these are the same thing—it's the same lacuna in the image the everyman, *le bonhomme*, has incorporated that stopped the hands from being able and deprived the other character of all help.

Thus, the film was perfectly clear. But how many viewers would have tolerated that clarity, would have watched—without flinching—those two hands at work for long sequences that were of course cut from other sequences, the others, regardless of what they showed, intercalated between them, and the viewer eager to once again find themself grappling with those hands for which tying a knot would have been the impossible masterwork? How many viewers could I assume?

Here one sees the difference between *camering* and making a film. The latter would be a question of providing the means with which to illuminate the pit so that one could follow the story and see the characters.

Whereas with *camering*, the means are lacking, or nearly so. That is, apart from the instrument, the video camera that allows one to '*videre*'[5] without much in the way of preparation.

To show two hands that aren't able to tie a knot is, without fail, to disappoint. That is why one must first deprive oneself, if only of the intention of being successful, of fulfilling the audience. Those two hands fiddling with the two ends of rope don't mean much.

But even though the film I'm talking about was 'realised'—that is, made by taking into account the reality it's assumed a viewer is capable of appreciating—and projected at the Festival de Cannes—the parallel section, not the commercial one—three-quarters of the viewers present, though well-intentioned, projected themselves out of the theatre after the first fifteen minutes. Even so, in the film *realised*, all that remained of that interminable sequence with the knot were trivial snippets.

As to the viewers' response of fleeing the outrage, why did one have it? And it's precisely that ONE was not having it, and in any case, the film was not for ONE; otherwise, the director, *le réalisateur*, would be *realising* what they suspect and assume to be the audience's reactions.

It's in this assumption that the director's convictions intervene—the idea they form, the judgment they make about their contemporaries. The director knows what to expect on their contemporaries' part. Should they be in doubt, distributors and producers will come along and fill in the gap through which what's new, what's surprising, could have gotten through.

For the vicious cycle of a film made based on preconceived ideas—I'm talking about the very content of the film, and the way it's filmed—to rupture, the director's intentions are not to be relied on, even assuming myself to be in that role, placing myself in that position.

The knot that isn't tied, that can't be tied, while the other kid croaks, clearly illuminates the reason he won't be pulled out of his pit. If Yves were capable of tying a knot, he would have done whatever it took for the other kid down there, who's like another him. But this him is lacunary—the proof being the knot that isn't tied—and so we know nothing of the other kid's situation. This event, which doesn't stop happening, which doesn't happen—and I'll leave it at that—isn't something I can assume I would have been capable of imagining.

It was unfortunate that none of us could use the shots taken, that we didn't have the money necessary to send the negatives to the laboratory, and we didn't know what we had filmed, if it was good, and visible, or completely black, or completely white, underexposed, overexposed, out of focus, or any of the other things that prevent images from being seen. Now, we took the precaution of filming—like there was no tomorrow, from every angle, at different distances—this tying of a knot that wasn't tied. And so all the images, all the little thirty-metre reels glued end to end, were the find revealed one year later. Which is in agreement with the words of Picasso: 'I do not seek, I find.' It's necessary to find first. That said, what's found still needs to be respected, which implies a certain disinterest in one's own intentions.

Now, when I frequented the cinema, what quickly seemed onerous and tedious to me was having to be subjected to the director's intentions. I would break out into a sweat and strain to see, in the images, the fleeting snippets that nevertheless got past, having eluded the *montreur*'s, the showperson's, intentional framing. More often than not, there was no room at all for them, nothing of the rest; everything had been willed, milled; what I had been taken for was clear to see and it was no laughing matter. There was misconception, if not contempt.[6]

To return to the other film that we have undertaken, *Mourir de rien*, what is it about? *Dying of Nothing*? Now, filming *nothing* is no easy feat. It's true the film is about a maniac, a person deemed irresponsible. He'll neither kill, nor kill himself. He'll die, of nothing; put otherwise, for lack of something. We'll see those with whom he spends his last moments. Whether these moments are his last, or his second-to-last, no one knows; himself included, no doubt.

But we'll also see his wife, the woman he lived with before being institutionalised, and this wife's close presences—'his' being a bit of a stretch in this case, an insane person having neither rights, nor assets.

Dying of Nothing. It would take almost nothing for him to live, to go on. Perhaps it all depends on her; perhaps it's all there. Perhaps this was determined *there*, and over a long period of time: a madman doesn't become one all on his own. And what is it that she's unable to do, that is not done, that was not done? What as simple, as obvious, as the knot in *Le Moindre geste* (*The Slightest Gesture*).

This entails a real find. Useless to search for it conscientiously. One must go about *camering*. It is perhaps by filming images and turning them into video that the *nothing* will appear.

One sees what it is *to camer*, in the infinitive, and what it means to evade the surfeit of intention that comes with believing the dematerialised image of the person reproduced like there is no tomorrow. The human, as I understand it, doesn't exist, doesn't take place in the frame of intentionality.

I remember another film: *Ce Gamin, là* (*That Kid, There*). A number of individuals aged twenty and older live close indeed to autistic children. If these children are *there*, then we are too, 'we' being some people who are not elsewhere.

Elsewhere? 'There', where these people would be if they were not *there.*

What I proposed was that the director film them not there—where they should have been—in milieux and places[7] that were easy to find because 'there' entailed where they were beforehand, before the attempt we filmed had been thought up.

The director was ready for anything, except having to film folks not there in the images he would take of the places-milieux where they had previously lived.

Yet 'there' was very much where the essential would be found.

If the children were not there, in the beds and places intended for them, it was precisely because we were there, and not in the previous elsewhere.

And 'there', *camering* should have taken place like there was no tomorrow in order to—perhaps—make the find: for their absence to become in some way palpable, even if only to the eyes.

What I expect of *camering* resembles dredging, if one understands it to be a matter of a chain with no end that's equipped with scoops that scrape the bottom. It's a matter of digging a channel in a port. Who knows what might emerge or remerge in the clarity of sunlight, provided, of course, that one takes a rather good look at the mud that surfaces, as though the project were there; that one looks around a bit, and not in the channel to be deepened. This is where the 'no end' that's necessary reappears—if one understands that a find is not a subterfuge.

Perhaps one needs to have experienced the school for autistic children to take the absence of intention to this degree.

It's here that the two attempts—allowing autistic children to exist and *camering*—have a trait in common: to evade intention, which requires a strange rigour that can't be intentional.

Camering?
It's a matter of the camera wandering; and it's by watching the images gathered that small finds emerge.

But if we have a film in mind, a project in progress, everyone who's filmed sees themself, foresees themself. ONE's gaze is always assumed. It's even partly what gives coherence to every-one-of-us: the other's assuming gaze.

It's no use going through with the subterfuge of everyone being able to express themself freely, even if only via attitudes and mimicry, as the 'self' and the 'one' are in close league with each other. The 'self' either conforms, or it provokes, which often leads to the height of conformism, which is termed novel, and there you have it, subscribing to the height of fashion being a good means of fulfilling a certain audience, while another part of the audience is frightened by this, always fond, as it is, of taking fright.

One should thus begin *camering* with folks who are not making a film. But then what are they doing there, in the frame?

It's hardly possible to *do* nothing, as this in part requires intent. And I fully understand that what's called for is the hardening up of a troop.

The space of an attempt is an *area*, a term that's familiar to us because an attempt is a question of residing as close presences with autistic children in living areas.

Does that mean that in and on the shooting area where camering would be practised, aspects of the *human* that eludes us would be revealed—aspects that are close to what there could be of the *us* in an autistic child's 'point of seeing'?

We can begin there, on the condition that we evade our inclination to similarise the other, whether or not they be autistic. Failing this, if we let ourselves get carried away with our assumptions—with what we assume of the other—there will be no rupture.

We'll thus need to find, specify, maintain a way to implement this rigour in our very practice—that is, to dam up our intentions. As to these intentions, we know their strength and cunning. The slightest fault in the dyke and they get through, with more fervour after having been contained.

And so, it's a refinding that moves towards a mutual understanding, and an effusion and recognition that would seem to be the minimum of requirements. But if everyone just winds up recognising themselves and finding themselves in the other, what's the use in working towards this? If it's a matter of putting out a new carbon copy of the same person as always, the viewer content as can be at recognising themself just as they were taught they are, the perpetual label that's the convention need only be affixed to the poster, whether the film is about love or murder, and off we go, round and round in that symbolic universe with no way out. Yet there are ways out to be found; they can be found. It's simply that they don't fall within the purview of perception. If they exist, they can be experienced by the inconceivable everyone. They are a matter of *émoi*, stirrings, which do not, strictly speaking, entail emotion, and so are not the convention.[8]

We're grappling with a shooting area in which camering is practised.

We can regard it as a mine.

A person seeking ore may be perfectly unaware of its usage, or rather the ulterior uses of the raw material detected by the sparkle of its specks.

Yet it's impossible to go about *camering* in the void.

To live and undertake the for-nothing mode, it's necessary to be autistic, and that's not given to just anybody. If we were autistic, taking a good look at the camera *qui tourne*, that's rolling, would more than suffice. It's quite common for autistic children to be drawn towards all that goes round, *tout tourner*. We might say '*moteur*' as we once said '*silence, on tourne*'—'quiet, we're rolling'. The camera would roll—*ça tournerait*—but as for '*action*', as we say, there wouldn't be any.[9]

It's impossible for us to act without a project's motor—what some might call motivation. As for action, it is needed. But rather than the end, it's sufficient for action to be the pretext.

Whatever we do, there is the act, just as we might say that while there is life, there is hope, hope for a different life that, as a miscreant, I fully understand could be taking place now. This life has always taken place, only we have not been aware of it.

This part of *the act* is liminal to everyone's intentions, whether the person in question be taking action or watching, and it hints at what there could be of a mode of living that is somewhat *human*.

In truth, this is the theme of *Dying of Nothing*, the 'nothing' being what's missing from the existence that has been given to us and which we would be mistaken in believing takes place *in* everyone. I want to talk about what exists *outside*—outside of this everyone.

We have a maniac who takes a psychiatrist hostage at gunpoint. The hostage will remain one for a few days in a place that exists as though it were a detour in what happens.

To tell the truth, nothing happens in this out-of-the-way place; put otherwise, nothing happens to pass through—not even information, the maniac having given the transistor a kick, thereby smashing it against a wall. Of course, some people are there, and among some people something always happens; all of the many remarks, small gestures, gazes that evoke the past and the future, which is literally unpredictable, impenetrable, opaque, though it may be very near. A maniac is there, he holds and has pulled a revolver.

We set about *camering* and filming prevailed—the requirements of editing were immediately visible, the film a finished product destined to be delivered to the other's gaze, the other projecting their influence on the images to be taken, the sequences always/already taken in that inevitable cadastre of measured time, the representation always/already there, inevitable, in all that presented itself in the camera's frame.

One is familiar with the double meaning of the word *present*, the Latin origin of which would appear to mean: push to the forefront.

Present: the person in the place, the group in which the person who's talking, or about whom one's talking, is found.

There is thus always/already a person who's talking or talked of in the place.

Where there is a person, what disappears is the human as I understand it: that which is deprived of taking place.

Present: action of giving something to someone; that which is given.

How can we ensure that what is given—to viewers—evades, even if only just a little, the omnipotence of the person who's talking/talked of?

This is one of the possibilities at play with camering: apart from the person who's feeling, believing, hearing, seeing themself, hardly *any things* are needed for the human to be there. These things are there; it's that they are not seen (by the self).

Every gift presupposes a pact, a recognition without which the person to whom the gift is given doesn't even perceive it, doesn't realise it, while camering seeks to create a gap in this very pact, in the agreement heard, even if it's only hinted at.

As to this 'agreement heard', we know what's in fashion: the glimmer of all those blinks, though rather than eyes it would be ears doing the blinking.

Attempting to free oneself of this influence implies not that doing so is a matter of liberating one's 'self', but rather something else.

Something else? That liminal human that we are not 'free' to perceive; though instead of free, it would be more accurate to say: not capable. We lack a sense; we may—perhaps—be well-intentioned people, fraternal and charitable, but as to the human, what's that?

A film needs a subject, while camering attempts to evoke what lies beyond the purview of the subject; whether it be the director or the viewer or that of the work.

We would appear to be at an impasse—the very impasse that is incumbent on us in the living areas where we reside close to autistic children.

There is no way out of an impasse; the space of an attempt would thus be, if not a way out, at the very least an indication that there could be one, and not one but a myriad; a Milky Way of sorts that is extraordinarily distant and, it seems to us, unattainable. Nevertheless, at times, in flashes, it's there, within reach.

But one needs an instrument, and a practice, and a director who doesn't place themself in the position of having to fulfil the viewer's wishes.

And the director's intentions are not enough. It's also necessary, if the director doesn't wish to produce a work of rubbish—yet another—for there to be pearls and diamonds, by which I mean real finds; there remains the mount, which is a question of workmanship, and design, taking into account the constraints of production and exploitation.

I happen to have written a few plays, the majority for marionettes, though at least one for the stage.

This was around 1943. Who knows what I might have been reading or what I had seen of those living in the area. In short, at one point, a certain number of individuals from the village in mind piled up in a pyramid; at its tip, an oddball exposed his rear end. I had perhaps been reading too much Claudel.

According to the director of a small theatre in Paris who considered—and why not—putting on my play, I needed to give up that moment, the one with the pyramid, since the stage's floor, no doubt a little weak, or rather worn out, or decayed, would not hold the pyramid's weight. I would have to make do with a single everyman who would show his rear end. Lost would be all of the effort involved in his climb up the heap of people to the very top. But it was at the top that he noticed the absence of the customary flag driven into the pediment of the highest of monuments; he was quite bereft, deeply disconcerted. Hence the summersault intended not to provoke but to hide the shame and distress he felt at being up there. And what then? He found he had lost his role.

I didn't respond to the theatre director. Incidentally, I didn't much care whether the play was staged. So why write it?

Why write a play showing two labourers the likes of which there must have been in the Middle Ages—artisans-companions whose work was to make coffins? They put so much creativity into what they did that those coffins were little boats or chariots without wheels. On seeing their work, one might have said they were making carousels. As a result, folks were more willing to die.

But death would not hear of it. The viewer saw death—a marionette, cantankerous, certain of her rights (and her duties). She came along and did so much grumbling that the two companions made her a proper coffin. Death, dressed in black, had come to carry out an inspection. One of the companions grabbed the old lady, tossed her into the coffin, and the two of them bolted the lid shut, the job done quickly and efficiently.

They were quite simply fed up of hearing her grumble. In fact, nobody in the region was dying anymore, which everyone eventually realised, even if it meant verifying what happened if, say, they cleaved their nearest contemporary's head in half with the blow of an axe. Said contemporary, though rather stunned, didn't die. The situation turned joyous; from joyous to riotous there is but a step. It was the latter that was more or less permanent. And so a young fellow came along and he was to have a trick: he needed only point his finger at one of the lid's nails for it to be struck from within by the bucks of death herself, and the nail to pop out. He thus held the power.

I must have thought up this short play in 1936 or 1937. I was a communist.

The nails popped out and every time they did one heard the air vibrate, as though it was being shredded by those little pieces of metal, which sounded like crystalline notes over top of the rumbling emanating from the oblong box.

This play was not staged either, as the person who had begun work on the characters never made it past the first. Now, considering there was to be a whole crowd of them up on stage, I figured it would be at least fifteen or twenty years before rehearsals could begin. A project that takes so long to be completed forestalls itself.

As a result, I eventually grew out of the habit of having ideas that were neatly arranged—I've no idea where—like plants in a herbarium. Realising them stirs up so many problems that it's best to take a different approach—a contrary one, as it were. I mean, to begin with what is, and not begin in order to leave, but to remain, there, to be there permanently, and by moving through what is, allow its self to be seen, the *self* never just being a point of view.

The fact that a point of view is rather unanimous doesn't prove that it should be trusted. One needs to go beyond a point of view to 'a point of seeing' that is no longer about the *self*.

I return now to *Dying of Nothing*, which is in the process of being camered; it's May of '79. What it entails is a madman who takes a psychiatrist and a nurse hostage.

Now, in day-to-day life a madman and a nurse are neighbours. They occupy their time as best they can. They talk. Suppose the madman doesn't talk, or nearly doesn't, what happens is that the nurse talks. He comments on the information as he hears it over the transistor in the cell-like room where the madman is often found lying on his bed. In the current climate, the taking of hostages is not uncommon. The nurse has some ideas. He expresses them. He comments whenever a blunder is made, each as large as a house. He makes the perfect hostage.

Now, we won't see any of this happen. We won't hear the nurse. Even so, it was a good idea for the news to seem like propaganda. With an external line, we grasp the reason for propaganda when it's a matter of advertising. But what about when it's a matter of the news? The propaganda continues, only the reason is not always evident. It's there like a lacuna. We talk of the exemplarity of being under pain—of death. What's needed is concern for the exemplarity of the very fact of information. But in both cases, who knows how things will play out.

In *Dying of Nothing*, the madman certainly seems to obtain a role, to suddenly grab hold of one, which is made all the easier because he has no other role to play, having been without one for quite some time. We might even believe he began to act the madman, bereft as he was, and lacking something else to do.

Having said this, one needs to be wary of good ideas. If one considers them to be good, one will want to illustrate them. And what happens with illustrated ideas? It's a sickening obscenity. It's as if the director had said: 'Do you see my intentions?' Well, yes; we do. And intentions are more or less always the same. So why impose one's view? Everybody has one. The filmgoer could say: 'Don't you want to see mine?' And this would be debatable—and interminable.[10]

If I don't place much blame on the other film we happened to make, *That Kid, There*, it's because of what I was told by those who attended its screening—here or there: they were surprised by the silence that followed. What could be more disappointing than a film about which there is nothing to say? Some might regard this as a major failure; to put it in more fashionable terms, as a veritable disappointment. And yet?

The space of an attempt is a space of rupture, even if only with what's in fashion.

I return now to *Dying of Nothing*. As to what might have taken place between the nurse and the madman prior to the hostage-taking, ONE will see none of it, or nearly so; a few snippets, perhaps, of the moment immediately preceding it. If I do tell what happened, it's because I'm telling it to those who will be the madman and the nurse—who are going to be them. And so *camering* consists, in part, of grasping the revelatory specks of those past moments that surface in this now that is in the frame. But this is one of the secondary tasks of *camering*.

The human, as I understand it, is not in the past, in history, in the life experience of everyONE.

It's what could be, at any moment.

And it's true that I'm always thinking of, and mulling over, films that are impossible *to make*—from the outset; otherwise, I would write screenplays.

A film completely impossible *to realise* would be one based on *Lord Jim*, the novel by J. Conrad.

A young officer in the merchant navy, the son of a pastor, a sense of obligation incorporated through and through, finds himself on board a cargo ship that transports emigrants—Malays I believe—as merchandise. It matters little whether they're migrants or pilgrims.

And lo and behold, the ship hits wreckage and is going to sink; it's a certainty.

The reaction of the ship's small crew is to save itself, to get away.

And Lord Jim, the hero, has no memory of having jumped from the ship into the getaway boat. He finds himself there.

He never saw himself jump. It's there that the entirety of the knot is located. Impossible to show this knot. If *one* sees him jump from the ship in distress, then he sees himself, and saw himself, jump. Everybody sees him, thus it's assumed to be seen, to be known, that he jumps, has jumped, has saved his life to the detriment of the idea he forms of himself and his obligation.

If one doesn't see him jump from the ship, the greater the knot. It's in this very act, which is not intentional, that resides all that follows in the story and the score to settle for the person unknown that is Lord Jim and all the others he goes on to meet.

There were perhaps several ground-up versions of this Lord Jim filmed, just as there must have been one or several of Moby Dick, the book by Herman Melville. It's obvious that grinding up the images around a theme—which is the case with many stories that have been filmed—results in the real theme being sacrificed from the outset; go try and film a white whale that one doesn't even know exists; what matters, what's the knot of Moby Dick, is the existence non-existence of this legendary whale.

This to say that what constitutes the real find in a story can't be the object/project of a film or one risks enslaving the images to nothing more than embroidery.

What's lost is the particularity of an art that has gone all the more astray now that talking has been thrown into the bargain—which consolidates the pact of the agreement heard.

What would the characters in Van Gogh's paintings say, the postman, the clown, the woman from Arles, the artist in his own rendering, Father Tanguy, the nude woman, the man with the pipe, if ONE had given them the word? A dire gift if we rely solely on what ONE contributes.

What did Van Gogh die of? It's true he killed himself, tired, perhaps, of not finding in life the art of living he revealed in traces in his works of paint, even if these were only fields of wheat, cypresses, and olive trees. He would have liked to be a pastor, but the language was not there. He was not able to incorporate it or—language helping with this—the attitude and the respect of conventions.

Hence the rupture, which incidentally was two-fold: in painting and in the infinitive, he broke his life.

I return now to the film we undertook around the theme: HUMAN/BEING.

After a few weeks, a few months, we saw the outline.

There is a necessary place, there is a milieu, there is an event.

A strange milieu that becomes one within the scope of the event of a film, so much so that it doesn't *really* exist. It has no reason to exist other than the film to be made, everyone representing the person they're assumed to be, this intention being more than a priority; there are no other reasons—the milieu involves re-creating an ambiance so that it will have a certain reality.

Now, as far as I'm concerned, there is reality—that which can be seen—and there is the real.

If the camera films a field of wheat under the sky and in the wind, it's reality that is thus depicted for us.

If the camera gives us images of a stalk of wheat growing, and if we see it grow, from that first growth, a sprout just barely pushing through the earth, and all of a sudden it springs up into a thriving ear of wheat that has weight to it, that is the *real.*

This real can in truth never be seen, while the infinitive, to grow, does exist. But go try and film an infinitive.

The artifice of image after image is needed, the first taken in April, the last in July. The projection would be one minute long. And everybody would be able to see that which can't be seen.

The camera as instrument positioned as though in a detour in time.

Here one sees the difference between camering and filming.

Let's return now to HUMAN BEING. There is the reality of the milieu, a place, and the beings who are conscious of being, and the reasons they're there.

To get at the real in the human, what's needed is a detour in which to position the camera: the artifice.

Otherwise, the folks that are there act out a story, each playing at being someone they strive to be as authentically as possible. I have seen films in which one saw Napoleon, Stalin, whoever you like—it matters little. And then I happened to see that stalk of wheat *growing.*

Filming the human should be possible.

The human existing, *l'exister humain*, is an infinitive in French, and to want to film it is to attempt the impossible. And yet it's here that the camera, and the camera alone, can make possible the subterfuge, the *detour* able to depict this *existing* as it depicted the stalk of wheat *growing* for us, the camera as instrument best fulfilling its purpose. That the human has no intentions doesn't mean it's lacking in needs. The 'needs' of a grain of wheat are numerous and varied. If it doesn't have what it needs—water, and earth, and sun—there is no growing.

Whether the folks gathered to meet the needs of filmmaking learn (what it is that's) their role or invent it matters little. Will they be/pretend to be characters who are more or less authentic? There is no doubt about it.

But what's authentic has nothing to do with the real.

That these characters are genuine concerns us. The human—the real—doesn't concern us, in the sense that it is not seen (by the self).

And this is precisely why one needs a camera.

Impossible to go about camering without a milieu that is not there for the camera any more than a stalk of wheat in the earth is. It's the camera that is there for camering, and not the milieu that is there—to be camered.

This requirement hardly seems manageable. To film the waves of wheat that ripple in the wind, one needs only an instant.

When camering is a question of a growing sprout, which takes place in an instant on the screen, months of time are needed, as well as a camera, immobilised, positioned in its detour, vigilant, on the lookout, attentive in order to respect the fact that the time period of the real is not that of reality, even though reality too will have to be evoked.

One sees the difficulty: seeing the human, which is real, as everybody suspects, and it being recognised if it appears, as though from below the surface. The rest of the ticket—that is, reality—remains to be seen, and not only the white strip where the real appears below the surface.

When we thought about making a film in which one would see a madman taking a psychiatrist hostage, the nurse being in cahoots, who knows why, the majority of those we wanted to play in it had been mad, or had been taken for mad, which amounts to the same thing; that or they had lived very close to others who had been labelled mentally ill.

It was easy to assume that those who had welcomed the mentally ill in their lives would be capable of playing at changing roles, of being the maniac, because they had lived close to others who were one.

It's not at all certain that viewers would have felt these folks to be more authentic if the role had been filled by actors taking on, so to speak, characters, which brings us back to those obligations and to what must be done.

I must have held on to quite awful memories from primary and high school for the word *devoir*, meaning both obligation and homework, to have forever after seemed suspect, to say the least.

If the actor—who does what needs to be done—is felt to be somewhat genuine, plausible, then it's he who supports a minor artifice. This involves nothing other than the changing of roles that is a constant in everyday life.

What if we get rid of the screenplay, the story?

We find ourselves with folks as they are, folks who in their lives have *welcomed* the mentally ill. Who knows why?

These folks have lived here or there, as best they could. And what happened to them is that a madman happened to arrive, a drug addict, drunk, depressive, schizophrenic, hysteric, or whatever else comes to mind. They accepted his presence, and on occasion it was almost a godsend.

As to their intentions, some of them could be seen. They were even expressed. They were what they were. They said what they said.

And there was the rest, which, incidentally, eluded them.

Why complicate matters?

Because the human is that rest.

Émile Copfermann, on reading the first thirty pages of this text written under the banner of misCREATING, said to me, 'Film absence? Intention—whether you like it or not—precedes camering. There subsists a linearity that is given by the camerographer. In filming absence, someone is necessarily present.'

So that's why we have never managed it, as though it were a question of a stupid bet. I said to myself that with an overstatement of that magnitude, no doubt something is bound to be true.

The omnipotence of symbolic domestication is unavoidable.

I often return to the Pentecost procession in the streets of Lille, to the parade of floats, small troupes of jolly fellows and giants, veritable monuments, and ambulant scaffolding cloaked in multicoloured fabrics atop which sat masques that were smiling and fuming, of characters legendary and familiar. Since I was very little, I had to tilt my head all the way back, or nearly so, to see their enormous mugs. After a while, the nape of my neck in pain, I once again looked forwards. And what did I see? The skirts of ladies and gentlemen—who had to don skirts in order to hide the carriage that transported the scaffolding. In the carriage under them was some everyman who bore, on his shoulders, the shafts on which everything rested.

And that is how I saw, in Gambrinus's red skirt, a small skylight, and in the shadow, the teeny little head of some old everyman. There was someone in there. He appeared to have a head the size of a fist. When I imagined the folks under the skirts, I broke into a sweat. I never went back to see the giants of the Pentecost go past. This is perhaps the origin of my foolishness when it comes to historical characters, who for many, seem to hold considerable charms.

In their absence . . . or rather in keeping them within the little skylight, framing them there, it's as though the character has become transparent and everything that happens to him can be seen. The monumental traces of history, and below the surface, the human, the little human who's in there, under there.

Perhaps he's proud indeed to play his indispensable role in the masquerade. Perhaps he could care less and is being paid to do so, since he's unemployed or works for the roads department and is putting in extra hours. Who knows? Perhaps while everybody is enjoying themselves he feels rather like a galley slave.

As far as I'm concerned, history, whatever it may be, is always monumental. Every character is monumented, and on parade: it's the Pentecost.

Is camering thus framing *in* the little skylight?

In or *through.* To see inside? To see from inside. Which is where the character we no longer see disappears. What remains are those who watch him go past.

Which reminds me that during the filming of *The Slightest Gesture* the camera didn't have sound. It took only images. And we could suspect that the sound we had recorded on a cassette player would never be synchronised. So then . . . ? What remained was to never put *whoever* was speaking in frame. Whenever someone was speaking, it was no less interesting to see those who were listening. All we needed to do was turn the camera around. Nothing was lost; on the contrary.

It's certainly the case that to film absence, a presence is needed. But one should not let oneself be misled.

Is someone needed to film a sprout of wheat growing? Only if that some one hardly expresses themself, which is the least that can be said. Thanks to the instrument, it's possible to see what is not seen (by the self), even though everybody suspects it's there.

Just like the unemployed man who breathed via the little skylight cut into Gambrinus's skirt. Everybody, all the onlookers, suspected he was under that skirt. Nobody gave him much thought, nor did they see him.

Can I say that—very little as I was—I had the intention of figuring out what was going on under there? Not at all.

It so happened that I had seen and that the image persisted; others would no doubt have erased it from their memory. The image would have been erased in order to keep the memory of the procession. Can I say that I voluntarily kept up this persistence, that I cultivated it? Perhaps I didn't have the sense of history. When one sense turns out to be somewhat deficient, the others are heightened.

It's very likely that I have never been able to read a novel as one should, or perceive a myth as is befitting, whatever that myth may be.

Now, the other day, I learnt something from one of the individuals who has been endeavouring at this camering that has eluded us: all of those who are rather attentive to what I may happen to suggest—or relate—are waiting for me to write a novel.

The novel having been written, the coast would be clear to attempt camering. A remark that at the time seemed completely absurd to me, though at its core was obvious.

In this remark, I found intact the paradox of the role that is incumbent on me in this network where one another live close to nonverbal children: to handle language as one lights backfires during a bushfire, thereby halting the momentum of the flames so they falter before going out on the already charred ground.

Having said this, Copferman's objection that 'intention precedes camering' needs to be understood. When it comes to the growing sprout of wheat, intention is limited to finding the detour of image after image, to keeping within it from April to July.

It of course remains to be thought that a human milieu is not a stalk of wheat, and that another *detour* must be found, one that will make it possible to sieve—to separate the bran from the flour; the bran being the everyperson who's conscious and unconscious of the folks in the milieu, what of their history and which of their intentions, conscious or not, are at play, and the flour is the human, who is not a tiny everyman that can be seen through a skylight, which is quite a pity.

The individual is not a tiny everyman who's rather hunched down inside the character he carts around. So then how many everymen must one think were under the skirt? Ten, plus one at the front, on the lookout, the pilot at his little window, his task consisting of keeping the giant well within the limits of the street and its crowned head from hitting the electric wires stretched taut right over the centre so the trams, then in use, could connect to the current.

This little group of eleven everymen makes up the individual as I understand it, and in this group, the shaft counts as much as the *one* in every.

To return to the film still suspended under the banner of 'HUMAN BEING'—still suspended in the sense that in being made, it's unmade—are the one or more marginal milieux that are its place more human than other milieux? On the fringes of a society, are the wrecks the best or the worst of what sinks?

One clearly sees that this is not the theme. To address it, one would have to assume criteria about the human, to trace a dividing line between what is human and what is not, or is less human, and thus have a point of view that is dominant, predominant, previous. Which is what Copfermann said to me: that we can't escape the *where* in which the camerographer places themself. Otherwise, where would the heart they need to get down to work come from?

For me, distinguishing the point of view from the point of seeing is a tired old tune, hence the necessity of that detour from which it's not a matter of distinguishing between the human and the inhuman, but rather of perceiving what there can be of the human that everybody suspects is there—the stalk of wheat *growing*—but that nobody has *seen*.

Nobody can place themself in the *point of seeing*; the camerographer, as a subjective self, is not there.

Could the camerographer be objective? It's the instrument that is. The camerographer's consciousness of being eclipses the real.

What remains is to attempt a use of the camera that captures aspects—liminal ones—of that *human* which eludes language.

Which is to say the distance that needs to be taken with what Copfermann calls the linear—words coming one after the other and marking the limits of a reality that is very often designated as having no way out.

For me, this doesn't entail the—previous—placement of what there may be of that distance, that detour, that artifice from which the camera could give access to the real.

It's a question of a find located *in* the very images that can be taken *outside* of the concern for intersubjective history.

This incipient find is not going to jump out at you.

Does it entail the viewer forgetting the camera?

On the contrary: it entails the camera being *there* to so great an extent that it's the camerographer and their intentions and their point of view that fade before the *point of seeing*.

And what can be said about this point of seeing other than that in living close to autistic children we place it as though it had emanated from a different memory than the one we have been provided. One of the characteristics of this different memory is the persistence of images. Everything happens as though what's taking place there, in the *moment*, in the field of seeing, doesn't prevail over what took place there yesterday, and on the preceding days, and during the months, and years, prior.

Whatever may have stamped this memory—in the past—leaves an imprint that persists and reappears, as though it were projected during the moment itself. And this 'image' that surfaces has priority, it prevails, and will determine *the act* to the detriment of what should be *done* because, precisely, in this 'memory', it so happens that time doesn't pass, or rather, what happens in and of itself doesn't happen in the *self*, but in another film.

Here one sees that *camering* is to challenge time, whether it entails the 'growing' of a stalk of wheat, or the 'welcoming' into a milieu that attempts to admit the other whose turmoil is such that they lack ethnic memory.

So then, what might human being mean?

In this greedy *point of seeing*, intentions are lost, whether or not they be those of the marginal; they are never just ours, by which I mean those of the viewer, taken to a bit of an extreme. In its unusual presence, it would seem that all sentiments of Christianity are devoured, or worse, that they nourish despondency or exasperation.

The milieu feels parasitised, threatened. It fractures into contradictory attitudes. One another no longer hear each other, in the literal sense of the term.

The thing is that it's insufficient to welcome the other as one would like to be welcomed oneself.

This changing of roles is out of place.

But then *what* can we bet on?

Camering should reveal clues about that *what* to us.

But the *real* is different from what seems like reality to us.

We need only think a little about the difference between being and existing.

Here one sees the ex, and the detour of artifice.

Notes

1 'Mécréer' was written in late May or early June of 1979 and first published in *Camérer. À propos d'images*, Paris, L'Arachnéen, 2021.

2 The French title is the neologism *mécréer*, 'to miscreate', which suggests the noun *mécréant*, 'miscreant' or 'unbeliever', so that for readers of the original work, it would initially bring to mind 'unbelieving' and then expand to encompass the meaning Deligny develops.

3 The infinitive *mécréer* is the banner over the French-language work. However, in English, it has been rendered as the gerund, 'miscreating', on several occasions.

4 In the French phrase, Deligny plays with the paronyms *manière* and *manier*, translated here as 'way' and 'to handle', respectively.

5 The French verb *vider* means 'to empty', and it is possible that Deligny hints at this meaning through the use of the Latin *videre*.

6 In French, Deligny makes use of the paronyms *méprise* and *mépris*, translated here as 'misconception' and 'contempt', respectively, in an attempt at approximating the visual and sonic effects of the original. *Une méprise* might also be defined as a 'mistake' or 'misunderstanding'.

7 Throughout the work, Deligny plays with the repetition between *milieux* and *lieux*, 'places'.

8 Deligny encountered the term *émoi*, translated in this volume as 'stirrings' and variations thereof, in the work of Henri Wallon and developed it further in his writings. He uses it to describe the response to images that rouse the viewer without aiming to do so. One is stirred in a way that is distinct from the subjective and psychological response that emotion entails.

9 '*Moteur, ça tourne, action*' is the rough equivalent of 'lights, camera, action'. *Moteur* refers to the camera's motor running for the take.

10 The French reads *'Et ça fait un débat(llage).'* Deligny's response to the question a filmgoer might pose contains a double meaning. Would we like to see their intentions? This would lead to both *un débat*, 'a debate', and *un déballage*, 'an outpouring' of said intentions.

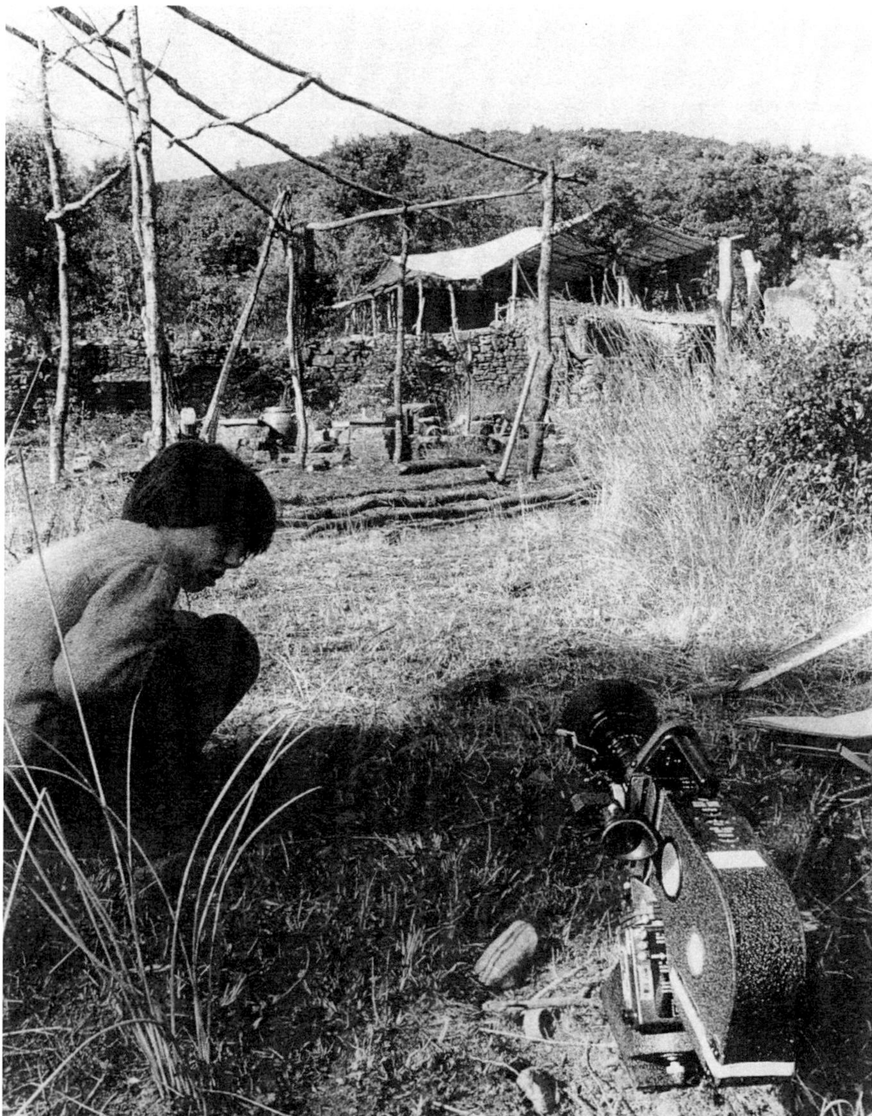

Benoît S. in the living area at Le Serret during preparation for the shooting of *That Kid, There,* around 1972.

Camering [1982][1]

1.

I just learnt, on the radio, that when Arthur Rimbaud, the brilliant rascal from Charleville, wrote 'le bateau ivre' ('The Drunken Boat'), he had never seen the sea.

What to make then of all he described in those verses that left their mark on the poetic art?

We need to tell ourselves that there is *décrire,* describing, and *d'écrire,* writing.

Is the latter writing from somewhere—from somewhere and about something?

I say this because the dictionary, which includes two written lines on the meaning of the word cinematography, cites, in italics, a bit of Jean Cocteau: cinematography is an art.

With Rimbaud, one sees what the art of writing can be.

There thus remains *camering,* and I have deliberately evaded filming, instead hanging 'to camer', the infinitive of a verb that—Still?—doesn't mean anything, as the banner over these pages.

I'm not a cameror.

I write; I live close to children said to be autistic. From where do I write? From there.

2.

From there, where I live, I see the world—like everyone else. It's not human.

From the sea, we have come. There was nothing, nothing but the sea, and then the bustle of it, and the algae and all the rest.

From the human, we have come. At first, there was nothing, nothing but a species that was completely unique, and now here we are, in both the here and now, certain of us equipped with a camera slung over our shoulders.

Chamberlains? The thing is that there would be a pope in the chamber.

Chambermaids? Then they would be waiting hand and foot on the princess.

Where Rimbaud had vocabulary, they have film. They have blank rolls and they have seen films; what they might connect is the earth to the moon.

3.

'To camer' is an infinitive, like 'to see'. For seeing to take place, it remains necessary for someone to look, so to speak. To go about camering, one needs a cameror of sorts.

If, having taken up the habit of writing, I can call myself a writor, that other person is a cameror.

Thus begins a change in direction.

As a writor, my culture is much older than that of the cameror, which appeared after 1900. It hasn't even been a century?

What can there be to an art that is barely fifty-odd years old?

There can be suckling, and though the camera gave birth to it, the nascent art can't suckle the camera.

When a mare is going to have a foal, her udders swell at the right moment.

As for the cinematographic art, wet nurses need to be found.

I'm talking about art.

What is an art nourished on?

On the milk of the art, at least at a young age.

4.

I happened to see, near Gravelines—where there now appears to be a nuclear power plant—a fisherman's wife give her offspring a filet of herring to suckle, the fish bronzed all over after having been smoked; it was not to nourish the child but simply so he could chew on something while waiting until the time came to suckle her breast.

Here then is the nascent art—which in my opinion, is far from having its first teeth—nourished on the milk of the surrounding arts: literature, painting, music. . . .These muses have generous breasts and it should come as no surprise that they fight to gain the newborn's favour; the small camera has so charming a name: poop, nana, rara. . . .The whole gamut. What will the camera get up to later on? It would appear that her father is light. . . .How about that. . . .

The daughter of light.

That's where things stand.

An art was born but not in the slightest because there was one missing from the panoply. Someone fashioned an instrument and there you go. . . .It remains to be seen what will come of it.

What's come of it, for the time being, is film, 'film' being the English word for *pellicule.* One places the *pellicule* inside the camera and out comes a film, which is screened in a larger box that is no longer called a camera but a cinema—this chamber being a room where people come to sit in the dark, or nearly so. There was a period in my existence when I spent most of my time in one of those rooms. I was initiated at a very young age. My grandfather, who was retired, often took me to a cinema called the Omnia. My grandfather preferred to sit on the balcony, in the first row of the balcony, so there would be no one in front of us. That is why I received a slap on the wrist of the hand with which I covered one eye; it's that I was farsighted and if I looked at the screen with both of my eyes, it was blurry—not the screen, but the images. Then, when I was older, I went time and again. I had glasses; the images were more or less in focus. Something was missing. What was I waiting for that didn't come? The slap on the wrist?

5.

The phenomena of nature, be it human nature, are not simple. Everything evolves and nothing should come as a surprise. From the origin of species to the origin of creative stirrings—it's an easy step to take. . . .

Let's pick up where we left off: my grandfather having died and my eyes outfitted with corrective lenses, my left wrist no longer had anything to wait for; no slap. . . .So if it's not the slap I'm waiting for, then what am I waiting for? I'm waiting for cinema to become what it could be: an art. . . .There would be no more asking ourselves if something were lard or pork, a novel or a work of theatre, a painting or a piece of music, industrial or artisanal, literature or who knows what. . . .Camering would exist like writing exists; we would say: the ninth (film) as we say the ninth (symphony).

I was talking about algae and the sea and the origin of humans, that is to say, of the species. No need to have seen the sea to write about it; the proof is that rapscallion of sorts who created a poem that may well be indelible.

He wrote it without ever having seen the sea. That said, each of the cells in the Arthur in question, who was poorly raised by a rather sanctimonious mother, no doubt hence the fact that perhaps creating, for him, was miscreating . . .[2] But I was talking about each of his cells, which are bathed—like mine and yours—in marine water with a salt content exactly that of seawater when life formed there.

Arthur, writor, wrote the poem, about the sea, without ever having seen it, but what does it matter? Eighty per cent of the water in that poorly coiffed chap with a head full of lice—if one believes the spouse of sir Verlaine—who was sloshed on absinthe, and you can see the eyes the old pal of poetry would have had: the sea, its mist, its languor; drowning eyes.

Camering?

Only a few moments of Rimbaud's poem and one sees the ocean; one sees it clearly, and this time, like never before. . . .Where did they get this from . . . (the camerors)? In the gaze of an old drunk.

And those who have no knowledge whatsoever of literary gossip whether it's old or contemporary? They have nothing to lose. . . .Someone could very well see through eyes that close like an oyster.

To do so is human.

6.

For a human being to have one oyster eye such that the image on the screen suggests that what they're seeing is 'something' *real*; something about which ONE can say to oneself: 'But is that the sea or what?'—this, without a doubt, is what *camering* is principally about. ONE says to oneself, and ONE can say to oneself, ONE can ask oneself, and ONE can even answer oneself.

But the cameror has not said anything and does not want to say anything.

Now, one might believe that emerging in these lines are the beginnings of a cinematographic art.

I have never touched a camera and would quite possibly get dizzy if I had to look through its small rectangular window. From where I see, it's a question only of *d'écrire.* And where do I write from? From there, where children said to be autistic live close by. Seeing them live, one perceives the existence of ONE, just as one would perceive the existence of the area the moment air is lacking.

ONE? The person, or rather, the consciousness of being *one*, in the world of people—which is what one is. Does ONE therefore only exist in this way? ONE exists such that one can question whether every one of us is something other than a single ONE.

I go see a film and it's some ONE who sees it. There is nothing else to see other than what one sees, and what one sees, one shows us.

Jean Epstein, a cineaste if ever there was one, talks of the 'revolutionary power' of cinema . . . because cinema is 'first a privileged instrument that, like the telescope or the microscope, reveals aspects of the universe that were previously unknown.'

One could not have said it better.

'From this moment on, cinematography (. . .) will allow for victories over that secret reality in which the roots of all that is apparent have *not yet been seen*.'[3]

'Moving pictures appear as though a universal language, a language of the masses, and a language of the great revolt.'[4]

The great revolt? It's about time. But against what? Against ONE. . . .

With the caveat that the cameror is a representative of ONE.

It's ONE who makes a film via the cineaste.

Are we no longer animals?

ONE is our species—or nearly so.

7.

Lacking a species—or nearly so—it's absolutely necessary for human beings to find themselves in ONE.

If they don't, human beings are immediately cut off from being a species.

They're not human; THEY are the ONE they are, even if only by virtue of their consciousness of this being so.

It's sufficient to see where ONE is—and there are films that show us, that send images back to us, of what ONE is capable of doing; it's useless to tell ourselves that *that* ONE is not *this* US. It so happens that this US has fully become ONE—it has happened, it is happening, it will happen; we will happen to become even more ONE than we were before.

Cut off from ONE, children said to be 'autistic' actually are one; would they, nevertheless, be of the (human) species?

They might perhaps be if the species still existed where we are; but where we are, ONE is too.

There remains camering, which would be seeing the human below the surface of the pervasive ONE.

Where would the objective, the project, of the great revolt be found, if not in awakening people to be less ONE and more human?

Bertolt Brecht expected this; he warned us; the human is on the horizon of a long conquest.

I believe he sought refuge in America and wrote a number of screenplays on commission—he had to earn a living—which could be found in the wastepaper bins of producers back then.

The great revolt . . .

If that is not the objective of camering, the camera does nothing more than grind ONE up.

So go on then and find a camera manufacturer and politely ask for a 16 or 35 mm equipped with a great revolt objective . . .

8.

The human only exists below the surface, that is why one needs an *instrument d'optique*, an optical instrument—though the instrument is not sufficient; it's entirely a question of the *optique*, or perspective, of what's also referred to as the point of view.

That said, the human is not seen (by the *self*); the *self* having, with regard the human, the eyes of ONE.

In other words, what's seen (by the self) is ONE.

What's seen (by the self) can be filmed.

And what about camering?

After I wrote the first lines of this piece under the banner of camering, images returned to me, intact, images from films, that are there, watchful, and that pester me: I'll have to talk about us. . . .

1947: I see a Soviet film titled *Road to Life.*[5] And I have seen the film, and seen it again, twenty times; I was the regional delegate at Travail et Culture and I escorted the film and was present every time it was requested. For months, I was *Road to Life*'s bodyguard.

Imagine the first images. Not long after 1917, gangs of vagabond children pillage, rob, and terrorise country and city, invading even the markets.

A small tribunal is created, established, formed, revolutionary men and women, the men wearing caps and the women headscarves. In the room, the smoke is so thick and so well filmed that it seems I can smell it. The kids who have been rounded up wait on the stairs and then start walking when one of them leaves the room, after having been tried.

The camera follows a peculiar fellow who is shaped like an Eskimo and has slanting eyes. The situation is serious. Peasants have been killed on the road a few kilometres from the city.

One of the kids leaves, stunned; the Kalmyk man enters; I'm almost certain, thirty-five years later, that his name was Burun.[6]

And there is a burst of laughter.

Imagine a good ten, perhaps twenty, Slavic revolutionaries bursting into laughter. . . .

Burun? The fact is that he reappears, after so many years, and every time he's tried and then he escapes, and then he's tried again, and so on, a stone skipping interminably, until it produces that glorious burst of laughter. But at the time we don't know any of this. There is the people's tribunal, the kid who enters, and the burst of laughter, and that laughter touches us. What was stirred up then, is stirred up again; it washes over me when I see those images anew; I see them, intact.

If the cineaste were to ask me what camering could be, I would say: projecting onto a screen fleeting images that will never be erased. Twenty years later, what was stirred up then will resurge as though a stone has once again been tossed . . . but where? Thereafter, over the years, I met a number of people who had seen the film. The same moment was always unforgettable.

The film unfolds, Burun becomes a Soviet hero who's killed by the counter-revolutionaries, his body placed in front of a locomotive, etc . . . etc . . . The history full of twists and turns, so to speak. There is the ONE that we are, to which we belong, and there is the stone that produces common stirrings. These images strike (us), but where? In the place that is common to everyone. There is the ONE that I am and there is what's common, reached only at the moment of being mortal, of which I'm not conscious.

But the cineaste is anxious.

Does camering thus require a twenty-year wait before one knows whether they have arrived?

What one says about a work of genius is true: only time is conclusive.

Does camering thus involve genius?

Of course, and yet that's the least of it.

Where then did the great revolt occur on that road to life?

It's there that we take on the crux of the matter, in all its difficulty: that of the director's convictional intentions and the meandering of History. Because there is History and there is the history of the brave Burun, vagabond, pillager, criminal, perhaps, and swapping gang for gang, he moves from that of the pillagers to that circumscribed by the pedagogical community of schoolmaster and the known result: a hero.

As for History . . . One need only imagine what I heard after 1947, when just saying 'communist' would put you in the position of a bottle at a funfair stall. The bottle would be encircled with a small necklace, each interlocutor armed with a good supply to throw at you: Stalin, Czechoslovakia, Hungary, Trial, Afghanistan, Poland, the Confession. . . .The confession and the whole system. The people's tribunal. The burst of laughter. Laughter, nothing but a burst of laughter that I experienced fully as common stirrings. That burst of laughter had to be lying around so that Nikolai Ekk—or one of the others he worked with—could pick it up and place it in the image mill that, incidentally, could not grind it up.

In the film, all that falls under the purview of convictional intentions is erased by History. What remains is the burst of laughter that incidentally doesn't mean a thing. Human stirrings.

Camering perhaps entails putting inside the camera, inside the box, human sparks like that burst of laughter, and that is all that can be found there, the common human, the sparks.

A writor, I have nothing more to write.

9.

That said, I believe that camering requires at least two people.

The writor takes care of the words, which one of the two must do, if only so the other's hands are free.

And it's a great privilege, an *aubaine*, a godsend, to have the hands free.

Aubaine comes from the word *aubain*, which simply meant someone who was not of the same ban; and when this *aliban*, who was from elsewhere, died, the seigneur of the ban would round up his possessions, hence *aubaine*.

To truly attempt camering, one must be an *aliban*. Some people are *alibans* from birth; others become them only after certain events have occurred.

They have to escape some from the ONE's ban, the dominant ban, the Seigneur's ban.

What a godsend to be free to go camering just like a child—or a halfwit—throws pebbles into the water, by which I mean into common stirrings.

As for the writor, the task is to write just like the grandmother's work is to knit while the boy is by the fountain, because the grandmother needs to be there so the boy can be there, and go about his work, so to speak.

The fact of the originality of the work remains. . . .

It's not the first time a boy has thrown a pebble into the water. Who said anything about the first time?

Once upon a time . . . Which is a way of saying that *that* time is unique; it's the first time and it's the last; it will never again be that time.

Once upon a time there was a people's tribunal. . . .

Notes

1 The second 'Camérer' in this volume was written in January of 1982 and published in the 2nd issue of *L'image, le monde* in the autumn of 2001. It was called 'Camérer #5' in *Camérer. À propos d'images*, Paris, L'Arachnéen, 2021.

2 On reading *mécreer*, 'miscreating', French readers would likely think both of the neologism 'to miscreate' and *un mécréant*, a 'miscreant' or 'unbeliever'.

3 Jean Epstein, 'Culture cinématographique', *Écrits sur le cinéma, Volume 2, 1946–1953*, Paris, Seghers, 1975.

4 *Ibid.*

5 Ekk, Nikolai, director. *Road to Life*. Mezhrabpomilm, 1931.

6 The name of the Kalmyk man was in fact Mustapha; he was played by Yvan Kyrla. Deligny likely confused him with a character from one of Anton Makarenko's books, the title of which is also *The Road to Life* in English and French translation.

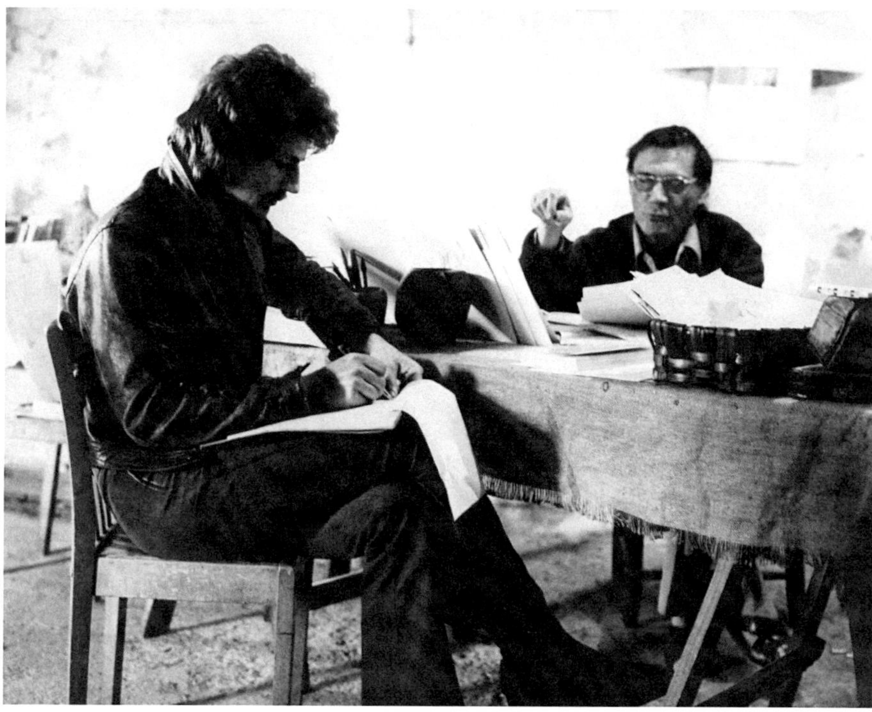

Renaud Victor and Deligny preparing for the shooting of *That Kid, There*, around 1972.

The Alga and the Fungus [1982][1]

1.

There are two of us, one writing and the other realising (a film).[2]

It's said that there is a literary art and a cinematographic art.

Between us, the question here is to find a way for the two arts to work together—with the utmost sympathy for one another, of course, but above all, in symbiosis. Lichen is a very hardy organism that has always endured, or nearly so; this little species of moss is quite obstinate and exists as a result of the meeting between an alga and a fungus.[3]

I believe that algae was the first to emerge from nature's breast; an alga is what I am, since writing had long existed when cinematography appeared; all of a sudden, along came fungi.

Between us, working together over the years will be a question of respecting the phenomenon of symbiosis, which is frequent in nature.

It will not in any way be a question of a union, or a designation, or something else that is overly conventional; an understanding is necessary; that we get on well.

What remains is to invent, between us, the workbench, which is not the oeuvre itself, but what the oeuvre will be placed on—between us; placed there, the oeuvre will be easy to handle.

2.

You happened to ask me for a screenplay. I evaded your request. You had shot the images in *Ce Gamin, là* (*That Kid, There*) . . . always without a screenplay. A series of images had been realised and these were in need of a binding; I thus not only wrote but said out loud what I preferred to call a legend rather than a commentary.

The years passed, and now here we are again, not with our backs up against the wall, but on either side of a workbench, or rather on either side of a space that is still vacant—a space where the workbench should be placed. It's clear that what we're missing could come from what existed during the shooting of *That Kid, There*. . . .: the living areas that existed for years; those in which the children said to be autistic resided.

We spoke of resuscitating a flock of kids who had emerged from the darkest depths of a cave.[4]

We got down to work. I wrote and you went about taking pictures of these—possible shooting—'areas'; all that remained was to imagine what would take place *there*.

The infinitive 'to imagine' should have put the 'understanding' bug in our ear.

To write the narrative I had no choice but to use my imagination; and so if the alga had done its work as alga, what became of the fungus? It had nothing more to do there; it became a girolle or a truffle or any other fungus that comes to mind; there was no more lichen, the lichen—the film—existing only in symbiosis. The cameror having left, the writor remained, with his story, his novella, his novel, or any other utterly linear form that comes to mind, at the risk of the reader, reading, imagining in turn—and freely, as it were. And the cameror being free to imagine a story, novella, or rather—and he'll decide for himself—a synopsis and screenplay.

3.

What one reads about cinema is surprising; just yesterday, I read an interview between Antoine Vitez, of the Palais de Chaillot, and Émile Copferman, editor of the *L'Échappée belle* series.

'Cinema has a lot in common with the novel. The art of cinema resembles the novel a lot more than it does theatre. . . .'[5]

Initially stunned, I thought: Why not . . . ?

I'll give you the book, though I did say to myself: – Let's hope the cameror doesn't take what Antoine V. said literally. . . .

To refute him, I'll talk about music instead—about music and painting.

For a number of years, a legend has been keeping me company; it's a legend I created all on my own, like a grown-up.

Two or three hundred thousand years ago, in the Amazonian jungle, there lived thirty or so indigenous people—their name or that of the tribe matters little. In accordance with their inherited customs, the tribe lived in an area they had cleared in the lush vegetation, and their shelter was a communal house with a roof that extended beyond the wall to form a canopy. Then along comes half-a-dozen indigenous people of the same descent with the same customs; they have had to cross the jungle; they have been walking for weeks; they're exhausted. They sit back against the adobe wall. Between them and the inhabitants of the communal house, there is nothing: no gesture, no sign. Everything continues as though they have not been perceived. Such are the tribe's traditional customs. What will happen in a few days is that they'll no longer be there, outdoors, but rather indoors, drawn in as though by osmosis.

But we're back on one of the days when the flock of newcomers is under the canopy, up against the adobe wall.

Some are lying down, others are seated, and a few are standing. One of the inhabitants leaves the house with a knife; it matters little if the implement is made of wood, stone, or iron. He approaches the newcomers. Anyone watching him could imagine how it might all unfold. But he is in fact going to trace each of their outlines on the adobe wall.

By trace, I mean etch in the adobe.

Then one fine day, the tribe abandons the living area. The roof collapses and the adobe wall falls, the etched surface into the earth. Now, it turns out that this earth has unique properties, among them, that of hardening the adobe, which turns to stone, or nearly so. Anything can happen in nature, and what happens two or three hundred thousand years after the brief event related here, is that an ethnologist, or an anthropologist, if you will, arrives. He rummages around and re-erects the section of wall. Why? No doubt because the anthropologist is not alone; he's with a whole band of porters and a guide and a scholar collecting scorpions. The fresco thus revealed is offered to the day and the public gaze. The adobe wall is transported to a museum that can only be the Musée de l'Homme and photos will ricochet in books and journals.

What I want to say to the cameror is that it's very likely that none of his films will draw the public gaze as much as these lines etched in adobe.

As far as I'm concerned, this is where the art of cinema originates.

One must not forget that *cinematograph* contains *graph*, while *cine* speaks of movement.

How can movement be graphed? This is where the real find is.

There thus remains movement—the optical illusion.

There remains *cine—ciné* being the abbreviation of cinema in French—which does a good job of showing what the—atrophied—word means: movement.

Le ciné reproduces movement; instead of a photo, now there's motion.

The graph having fallen like dead leaves fall.

Between the writor and the cameror, where to graph? Because it's the *where* that doesn't take place, the *what* being only of secondary importance, given the fact that it comes second, and only intervenes in second place.

What remains is to find that which comes first, the primordial.

It's the workbench I'm talking about here—the easel, the staff, the page or any other support that comes to mind; that is, *what* supports.

Once upon a time there was a little duckling that couldn't swim. . . .

Quite simply because there was no water.

Swim . . . On what, in what . . . ?

Graph . . . ?

Antoine V. tells us what *cining* can be based on: the novel.

The novel may make filming (*cining*) possible. There is movement, feeling, suspense, and anything else that comes to mind.

There remains *camering*, which I have written as the banner over these pages; *camering* would be a question of 'tograph' rather than the term in use, '*ciné*'. I think of it as a stump of sorts: the arm that is seen lacks the hand. Would the hand have been cut off? If so, by which fanatical power?

4.

There was a time when I went to the cinema; the cinema went well with me. This was before the war—the last one—on rare occasions during it, and for a short while thereafter. And then never again, which thus takes us back thirty or thirty-five years.

1981/1982; the military in power in Poland, Stalinism, Sovietism, Brezhnevism . . .

During the time that I went to the cinema, and the cinema went well with me, I saw a Soviet film: *The Road to Life*, based on the work of Makarenko, a Stalinist educator;[6] I was a young communist then, and had been since 1933. And while I myself was grappling with young delinquents, I saw this film and some of its images struck me to such an extent that from then on, a keen-eyed observer would have perceived its imprint in my attitude.

I can attempt to describe the images that struck me: – The film is about vagabond children who pillage the market and rob the peasants, wielding clubs and razors, and forming wandering bands. Every so often, there is a raid and a few dozen are taken to prison and come before a sort of tribunal that will decide their fate. This tribunal is a people's tribunal. When was the film made? 1927? Some men and some women are smoking tobacco and one literally sees the smell; a kid, with the stature of an Eskimo and slanting eyes, is summoned. The fact is that he's being summoned for the seventeenth time; he's caught, escapes, is caught again; a recidivist, he's dangerous; his gaze evades the gazes; and, in the tribunal, there is a great burst of laughter; *him* again. . . .'You're back'. . . .The Slavic spirit, Gorky, the justice of the people; he'll become the film's hero and will die, killed by counter-revolutionary brigands. What I want to make clear is that these images are not erased. Everything that I have been able to understand, learn . . . Nothing has been able to erase this imprint. I insist because this is what *camering* entails. In the blink of a camera, a bit of human.

It may seem like I'm saying that the members of the tribunal were more human than the representatives of our justice system in 'capitalist' countries; I may have had this thought; I may have said it to myself; though it's true I have never seen—not from close, nor from far—a tribunal in Western Europe. The revolution over, the Soviets weren't stiff in their roles as tribunal members?

Indeed . . . The striking fact here is no doubt that ONE expects something . . . and another thing happens; one expected a sentence; there is a burst of Slavic laughter, the women in headscarves and the men in helmets. In truth, the Mongolian kid is a clown. ONE can't judge a clown; ONE can't, and not because one shouldn't, but because it's humanly impossible. I fully understand what's outdated about the 'cliché' glimpsed here; I understand it all the better because I insist: It's a ploy, an imposture, a trap. . . .It's entirely possible; I'm not certain; nothing will be able to persuade me that the *human* was present during this moment. No doubt, I said to myself, the human was not present until after the October Revolution; but what I said to myself matters little, as does that which Nikolai Ekk, the film's director, its *réalisateur*, said to himself, or wanted to say.

Is it Ekk who we owe for that scene, that moment? But then *who* do we owe for the etched lines in the adobe I spoke of earlier? And why does it matter to us what the indigenous person armed with his knife or a sharp stick *wanted* to do?

Why does it matter to us what the painter, the composer, wanted to do, what they said to themself while they created their oeuvre? Every oeuvre that persists involves as much chance as did the fresco etched in the adobe, the first surface to fall into the humus of the Amazonian jungle.

5.

And this is the clearest thing that as a writor, I want to tell the cameror.

The cameror must give a good deal of consideration to the light.

He knows this.

And I tell him:

– Treat chance as you do the light: with the utmost respect and even a bit of fear.

The camera's mechanisms do nothing other than accept light. The billions of synapses in the cameror's head have the essential task of accepting chance. But if there is a possible analogy between chance and light, it's that while one needs both, one need not have too much of either; film, that thin layer of skin that appears to be dead, is very sensitive.

From the froth of gossip that forever coats biographies, the rumour reached me that Makarenko became furious on seeing *The Road to Life*, even though the film really was about his life and his oeuvre. Which goes to show there is a margin between the writor and the cameror; the alga and the fungus; symbiosis and non-intention and confusion.

Accept the exact amount of chance needed at the right time and there will be human in the images, it being obvious that *human* doesn't mean anything. What the cameror must really be wary of is what ONE means to have the human say.

Those who speak of art speak of creating, a majestic word if ever there was one.

Camering is miscreating.

There is the writor and the cameror; it is thus between them that camering will be established, which comes as no surprise, since the human only appears below the surface *between* one person and another.

As to what *is* there—that which is subjective and what the everyperson might want: Why would we give a damn about that? And yet it's what everybody is interested in. . . .It's hard to believe!

But art is not what ONE thinks it is.

Just look at the allure of the sea for the common person. . . .The common? Better to say one person and another who to the sea do go.

That said, take Arthur Rimbaud's 'le bateau ivre' ('The Drunken Boat') and tell yourself that while Arthur wrote this indelible poetry about the sea alone, he had never seen it. The boat that returns in the last lines, after its stormy journey, wrecked in a puddle in its home country, is Arthur; this is just about the only part of the story that's true.

There remains *the common* and the allure of this poem for the innumerable readers who can say (to themselves) that they have it in common.

What is the relationship between 'le bateau ivre' and camering? None; if there were one and camering were to take place on the basis of, apropos of, Rimbaud, and if I were the writor of this undertaking, I might forget the poem; there remains Rimbaud, ten years later, something of a geographer, a vague explorer, and in a precise way, the trafficker of weapons of war; he's limping low, like an invalid in the Commune, and at this stage founds a small school, while below the surface, one glimpses that he's written—who knows where or when—'le bateau ivre'.

Does this mean that a phantom boat should appear on the screen? Not at all; definitely not; the common person has no culture. Then what do they have? A certain innate sense of the human. This man with a limp, the survivor of a war to which he arrived late, barely understands the language of the slight indigenous people gathered around him. There are a few gestures, a few looks, a few mimes; also the light, at that hour, at the desert's edge; and the mountains that move past the horizon; and chance occurring when the camera shoots; the images unforgettable. As the writor, I'll tell the producer that the film is about a 'Life of Arthur Rimbaud'; if the producer doesn't know who he is, they'll look him up in an encyclopaedia, and a lot of people will come, even if only out of mockery, to see what we made of the life of a great poet whose mother was a staunch believer and who Verlaine shot—not the mother, but Arthur.

6.

'Show me your screenplay. . . .' says the producer, and they have a point; if they've got to place a wager, they'll want to see the nag. . . .

– He only has three legs. . . .

– Of course; that's what makes him original, as it were. . . .

– Original? What I want to know is if he'll win. . . .

– Right, but people are used to seeing four legs on a horse. . . .Mine only has three. They'll come see him. . . .

The producer pricks up their ears. . . .

La mère d'Arthur Rimbaud, the poet's mother, was quite devout; as for *la mer*, the sea, Rimbaud had never seen it when he wrote the chef-d'oeuvre on which it's based; yet when it came to *sa mère*, his mother, he was unable to see her.

What does the writor play? I'm not sure what the writor plays but I do know what they play with: words.

And the cameror? With images? Not at all. With chance. The cameror tells this to the producer:

– Chance is going to be playing. . . .

– Who?

Piccoli, Mastroianni, Dutronc, de Funès . . . de Funès as Verlaine? What about Rimbaud . . . ? A transvestite? The producer has to prick up their ears whenever there is gossip that might be of use.

– You were telling me about the weapons. . . .Was he going to sell weapons down there . . . ?

Yes, that too. It's not bad . . . it'll make for a screenplay in the end—the weapons that Libya or Iraq or Lebanon or some other place sells down there. . . .As for the viewers, it'll tell them something. . . .Because the producer yearns to be a scriptwriter, and it eats away at them a little, while the scriptwriter yearns to be a (great) novelist, and it eats away at them, and the novelist, if they have managed to stick around long enough, wishes to be a poet, and there you have it. But what about the poet? Here he is, a weapons dealer in Abyssinia or something to that effect. . . .There remains the story of the drunken boat . . . that appears in the soup like a piece of fat; the poet turned weapons dealer . . . his cargo ship sinks, 115 or 130 minutes pass, and then he's in a boat, and all that's left is to decide whether the Arthur who has been biographised is the drowned man descending, pale-faced, into the Abyssinian abysses, or if he survives, a Bombard of sorts, cradled in the very breast of his immortal dismasted symbol.

Now, this scenario is no more absurd than many others, and camering can occur like shells destined to the underside of the hull of any old story. . . .

When I was a (film) critic for a magazine up in the Nord, I went to screenings and watched movies; it so happened that the most idiotic of them were the richest in moments that touched (you)—But where? But what? All these—inadvertently human—'moments' lost. . . .Just like in life.

What about art—that of cinema, in this case? Bertolt Brecht, speaking of the theatre, warns us: The human is what's at stake in a conquest that is obstinate, slow, precarious. . . .

Camering is mis-creating; that is, not believing what ONE considers a human being.[7] But is not believing *this* enough? *This* being the Person just as they wish to appear? Not believing this is not enough, and not only is it not enough, it's literally impossible. Not believing this assumes and requires another *this* that would establish itself in the place of the *this* in disuse.

What about the creator? Which one—the creator with or without a capital 'c'? And just so you know, it matters little; they're one and the same.

7.

Is it the writor or the cameror—the alga and the fungus—that has language?

At first sight, it's the writor who makes use of it.

But if the human is always that which can't be said, when it comes to mis-creating, the miscreant will largely be privileged.

Notes

1 Deligny likely wrote 'L'algue et le champignon' in 1982, though it was first published in 2021 as part of *Camérer. À propos d'images*, Paris, L'Arachnéen, 2021.

2 Here and elsewhere, Deligny uses the French present participle as both an action taking place and a neologism for the person who acts: *écrivant* is both 'writing' and what has been rendered as 'writor' in English; *réalisant*, both 'realising' and 'realisor'.

3 Though in the past lichen was often referred to as a moss, it is no longer considered as such. The latter is a simple, one-organism plant, whereas lichen is a combination of two or more organisms that live together in a mutually beneficial relationship.

4 Deligny is referring to a fictional film project titled *Peaux d'argile*. Its manuscript is stored at the IMEC.

5 Antoine Vitez and Émile Copferman, *De Chaillot à Chaillot*, Paris, Hachette, 1981.

6 Nikolai Ekk, director, *Road to Life*, Mezhrabpomilm, 1931.

7 In French, Deligny's neologism, *mé-créer*, translated as 'mis-creating', also hints at 'un-believing'.

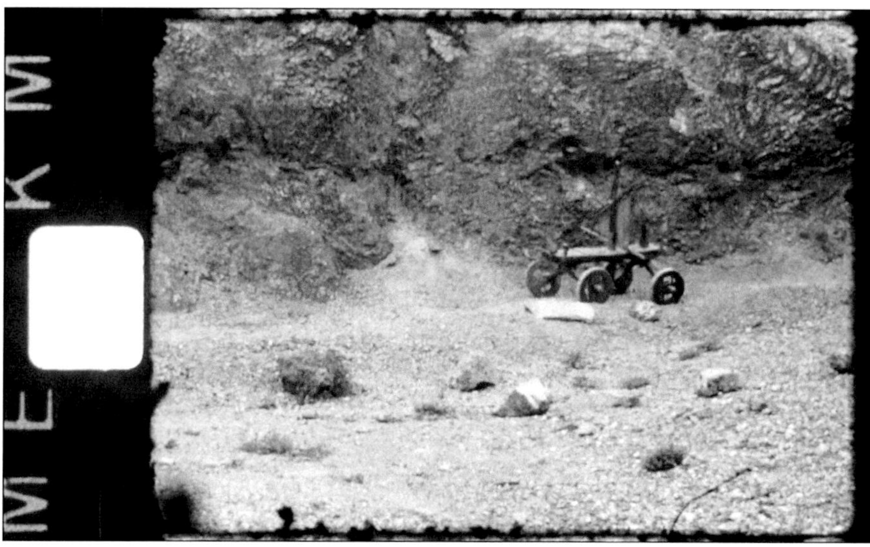

Shot taken with a Super 8 camera by Jacques Lin for the film project *Malabur and Pipache*, around 1982.

Fossils Have a Hard Life: Apropos of the Image [1982][1]

1 - To begin by saying that images are not seen (by the self).

Image takers visit me here, on a regular detour in their paths.

They leave their contraptions someplace else—I'm not entirely sure where—such that their hands are to be found at the ends of their arms, their hands, and there you have it.

They're not very old; I am.
I tell them stories, stories full of images. They can't take the images; it's not that I prevent them from doing so, but that the images are illuminations. They have a camera. They need images that move.

What I say to them is that the images they seek are on the screen, just like a painter's work is on the canvas. There is the canvas; that's where the painting is. It's not seen. It waits, and always will. Painters have said this. No one believes them.

This is what I say to the image takers:
– 'Images are not seen (by the self).'

This hardly helps them make progress; how can they take what is not seen (by the self)? They're not out of the woods yet.

I tell them the story of a mate of mine.
He and I were the same age. In 1937, I found him sitting on the floor of the small flat I lived in, its window opening onto the Place d'A.,[2] the square in a small town in the Nord of France where there was an asylum and I was the teacher at this asylum. There was a class of children who were slow. I told them stories.

I had lived with the mate who was sitting there, right under the window, his back against the wall, for months and months among the dunes by the North Sea. He had enlisted in the Brigades and gone to Spain. And as for myself, I taught children who were slow.

There was a jocular air about him, as always, which didn't hide the fact that he appeared a bit weighed down. He said to me:

– 'It's nearly finished over there. . . .'

I thought he had come to stay. He told me he was an officer and that he had been wounded three times. It's one thing to live among the dunes by the North Sea, and another to live two to a small flat, its window opening onto a square with a belfry, and the little bell in this belfry playing a few notes of 'La Madelon', just enough so one can recognise it.

He took a plump wallet from his pocket, a meek look on his face, like a turtle. He rummaged through the papers, the cards, the bills, the photos, and pulled out a small scrap of something that was neither cloth nor paper, something greyish-white in colour, rectangular, almost square, the size of the palm of one's hand, and he placed it on his knee. It looked like he had a patch on his pants. He said to me:

– 'It's the priest's skin.'

This as if it were nothing more than a billet of invitation.

And he told me that the priest had been in a tree next to his presbytery. In the garden, there was a well, and it was the only well in the village that still held potable water. All the other wells had to be poisoned by Franco partisans and the priest had killed those from my mate's unit who had come in search of water from the well. The bodies were still there, near the well, and my mate said:

– 'We did him in. . . .'[3]

He set out for Spain again. Who knows what became of him.

The two image takers never stop by together. When a story has returned to me, I tell it willingly, and each time I do, it's not exactly the same; as a result, I don't get bored. Each time, the story surprises me; it returns to me; it's the same and it's different.

Once upon a time there was a citadel named Vauban, after the man who designed the plans, and all around it, there were walls, walls everywhere. Between these walls and the Canal de La Deûle, there was a vast field that was vacant and bare, after having been a parade ground. Military parades had become fossils. In their stead, during the month of September, funfair stalls, carousels, and circus tents sprouted up. One would have to believe that the military parades of times past were particularly fertile.

Stalls of all kinds covered the esplanade. There were even stalls across the canal. To get from one side to the other, you had to take the Pont Napoléon.

At the age of six or seven, I was already quite afraid of crowds. In the morning, the esplanade was deserted, or nearly so. It was then that I went. I went to see the stalls. I only ever really saw planks and tarps, though on one morning, I saw a little monkey in a parrot's cage hanging from the pediment of a stall.

The image takers visit me in a room that's a regular detour in their paths. If the room were that of a guesthouse, I know what would be on its sign: – a monkey in a parrot's cage.

Since that morning, I have known what the human person entails: a monkey in a parrot's cage. I feel a certain sympathy for monkeys when I see them from a distance and feel far less for parrots, in particular because of the squawks they emit that remind us of language.

This citadel has seen it all. It's there that I received my war uniform in '39. And it's also there that one good fellow, *un petit bonhomme*, among others, who would have been going on sixty, was shot. He would not make it that far, having been shot like a hostage, and a hostage because he was a freemason.

In 1930, I didn't know he was a freemason. I saw him arrive, almost every day, in the courtyard of the school where only our class was waiting for him. He was always late. He would stand in the middle of the courtyard and swing his watch by its chain and the chain was long enough for the watch to become a pendulum. The good fellow looked at it perhaps to see if the earth was still rotating in the same direction. He taught us what thinking means. He was done in.[4]

What's the moral then?
If he had been in my shoes in '37, or rather, if the mate who had returned from Spain had been one of the students who stopped by to see him again, on a detour in their paths, what would the good fellow have said when he saw the priest's skin, like a knee patch on a pair of pants?
Would he have said:
– 'Go put that back where you got it from'?

But the Brigades' watchword was that they would not pass, that they must not pass, and those who did pass, would do so in around '40 such that the good fellow would be shot, which was a matter of chance, since he could have been transferred someplace where lampshades would have been made of his skin.

One after the other, the image takers nodded their heads.

Each would have closed their fists when the time came. Now, their hands are to be found at the ends of their forearms, which are resting on their thighs.

Here they are, the image takers, and I tell them stories when they visit on a regular detour in their paths.

To make a film, you have to take images. So off they go, to take images. When they return, they tell me there aren't any. They haven't seen any. I respond that there are images everywhere. One of them says to me:

– 'Are they fossils?'

Because fossils are also everywhere. I told them this, I even told them that fossils had a hard life. The old monkey does what he can in order not to speak like a parrot. He's quite content when he manages it.

2 - Art is a fossil in the spirit of the times.
Art has always been in *l'air du temps*, and always a fossil.

How is art made? Once upon a time there were two neighbours who lived next door, or practically did, and didn't know each other; fate—or whatever you want to call it—had housed them in the same part of the same town, which was almost a faubourg. One was called Laurens and he was a sculptor; the other was a painter and he was called Braque. Braque's wife was a childhood friend of Laurens' mother, and Laurens had suffered from bone tuberculosis. Who knows what of the human might have unfolded between these beings. The sculptor's son is the one to relate that his father, who was not a chatterbox, said: Every sculpture is in the air, *l'air*, but comes from the water. It's a simple idea. They lived in poverty but didn't speak of it, because in that part of town, poverty was as ordinary as can be. What's more, some of the townspeople were poets. There was, and still is, art in the two neighbours' work, and there you have it, that's all that can be said.

Their work was human and the human is a fossil in the spirit of the times.

This is what I say to the image takers:

– 'Fossils have a hard life. . . .'

Fossils have every likelihood of disappearing, from one generation to the next, and lo and behold, through ashes and ruins, they reappear, ironical; they don't do it on purpose.

This is what I say to one of the image takers:

– 'The Hercynian belt—it being where we are—was under the sea a few hundred thousand years ago. Images—if there are images—will come from down there, where the sea has only just retreated. Few are those who have heard the Hercynian sea spoken of. No need to know of something in order to see it. To see what? Images. But images are not seen (by the self). No need for the *self* in this adventure. 'To see' is an infinitive that exceeds and largely overflows what is seen and can be taken (by the *self*). If there is human, there is image. Now, the human is everywhere, in every head and likely a refugee in the unknown hemisphere of our encephalon; the human retained because it wants nothing and doesn't even know that it is "it", refractory as it is to identity.'

That said, the image taker knows full well that what's involved here is the making of a film, while camering is endless, and if he's got to make a film, he'll have to concern himself with being popular.

The image takers are entirely in agreement. Cinema is a popular art.

What I say to the image takers is that contrary to what is said, they don't have the images in their heads.
The images are in the spirit of the times.

The image takers could be poachers. They would get to know the images' customs and uses.

I'm thus a regular detour in the image takers' paths, and I anticipate what one or the other will say to me when they visit:

– 'I don't give a damn . . . I take it slow, I avoid the wind when it picks up, I hide my camera, and I don't give a damn. . . .'

I anticipate this and I know how to respond. I'll say:

– 'The shade of *one* . . . You head out and you think you're alone; you only see what's seen (by the *self*); in front of you and without your suspecting it, the shade of *one* is extending; now, images have an instinctive, innate fear of this shade. The human is refractory and *one* wants to seize it, assimilate it; *one* wants to make others believe that it is the human, while *one* is Man as he is. And what can happen is that Man believes himself to be—or wishes to appear—human;

> Man does what he can towards his fellow beings, *ses semblables*; *semblable*, similar—the human is not a similar being; hence the savagery of images. Whatever you are, whatever you want, you give to *one*. The shade of *one* is your shade in person. And regardless of your intentions, images can't be relied on. But what does this matter? You head out. If there are images in the shots taken, it's *one* that is perceptible; you perceive the stirrings returned to you; common stirrings; what's more common than the human?'

And I'll go on to say:

– 'It's enough to think of two gravities: that of language and a different one; images are of a different gravity than that of language.'

In the cinema, I saw an ant run across the collimator sight of a machine gun. Image. The film was by A. Malraux.[5] It was about the Spanish Civil War. Images don't mean anything. Nor does the human. Be that as it may, what mattered to A. Malraux, who had gone to war in Spain and had gone about making the film, was this image. Who would believe me?

At the very least, those who find themselves going to war, so to speak. And one can clearly see that this is a matter for the cinema; at the theatre, one would not see the ant; on a sculpture or painting, the ant would not remain for long. Because it's not a matter of capturing this ant, of capturing it in the canvas primer, nor even of saying, if we were at the theatre: – 'Look . . . an ant . . . ' Here, too, the ant would be captured; *one* would comprehend this; in the cinema, the ant runs, very much alive, which is completely preposterous, and completely indispensable; nothing is more necessary than that which chance alone can do; and in the process, the human recognises that to which it owes its existence.

3 - Might the image takers be individuals without intentions?

Certainly not, even if their only intention is to make a film, though there are others, and among those others is the pressing need to live in a network.

Nothing more human than living in a network.
I happened to say:

– 'If our project is to make a film, who knows if what counts isn't the network that thus weaves itself?'

The individuals find themselves a place apart from the rest; it's their atelier; they shut themselves up there. That said, paths weave themselves through their surroundings, in the same way that a spider's web weaves itself. It's a fossil, this spider's web of human networks as ancient as the hand.

Now, these networks exist, would exist, do exist, without one knowing it; there is no need to will them into existence. Who could be made to believe that if a spider spins its web, it does so to trap flies? No one. And yet everybody believes this to be true; *one* says that a web makes it*self* and the *self*? It's the spider.

On the basis of which, *one* comprehends nothing about nature.

Now, the human I speak of is nature; all that lives has a certain gravity; people have created a different gravity through the fact of language.

There remains the primordial gravity through which images exist.

Between the two gravities, there can only be coincidences.

This is what I say to the image takers:
– 'Images are coincidences. . . .'

They're willing and eager. It's thus a matter of creating canvases that will lend themselves to coincidences.

Camering is endless in the sense that the image taker can't will coincidences to occur.

Wider detours than those of science.
Camering requires different detours.
There are images that strike us and a good many of those who make films think they can will striking images—that they can will them to be made, to be taken, so to speak; and then nothing is astounding, appalling enough—the pictures are a display of atrocities that would like to be surprising. Images never strike in this mode. What's seen in these shots that are undeserving of the name 'images', as they are not at all of the same nature, is the manufacturer's intention, and nothing else; what's seen is what the manufacturer wanted to make seen. Is this obscene? There are times when one appreciates obscenity, which is a matter of language, not image; of audacious language users and no one else. If one really wants to talk to this subject—the language user—about images, one might say they're akin to fowl that have long been domesticated, and that are fattened up, deformed, weigh a lot—fowl that are made and cultivated for this purpose. Images don't have wings, but if they did, their wings would have

long been rendered useless and been in disuse and even been quite superfluous. One really has to wonder what a laying hen's wings are for. And if cows had wings? Not a problem, as long as that their wings don't inconvenience milking. It's well known that cows' tails are already inconvenient enough. It's even quite surprising that good dairy cows don't have short tails. Nature resists and persists despite everything.

But it's easy to comprehend that the 'images' in cinema don't resist culture. They have neither tail nor horn—nothing; they are views, Visions; which is just what the excellent U.S. of A's factories have, thanks to the 'know-how' of thinkers the likes of Henry Ford. Everything is made in this mode, including images. And as a result of the intensive production of armament, 'we' managed to defeat the Nazis. Would images thus be arms? You had better believe it. What about the resistance? Strange guerrilla warfare that. Except that we don't give a damn about the enemy's arms and though the camera may be an impressive arm, it is one only because of what it projects. Take the crew of a bomber—an 'inhuman' job if ever there was one, that of wiping out towns, hamlets, with bombs; and yet among the crew members, the human exists. Tireless spider that weaves wherever it is that people are in need, and in so primordial a manner that what is woven eludes them. Nevertheless, as to what could exist of the human among the individuals that form the crew of a bomber, the least that can be said is this: what they project is not there—that which, in sum, is projected; the projectiles are packed full of whatever you like, except for the human, which escapes being 'dispatched'.

Fossils have a hard life.

According to anthropologists—and I believe them willingly—from the start, the human being has thrown stones due to the fact that they stood on two legs, allowing the other two to be free. In those days, fearsome predators were not lacking and there was nothing fearsome about human being, who could not scratch or bite, nor even flee quickly or take flight. And lo and behold, by throwing stones—*jeter des pierres*—human being more or less managed to survive.

Fossils have a hard life; people still throw things; they have found better things to throw than the stones they gather, and catapults other than the hands at the end of their arms. What remains is projecting, *projeter*, the 'ject'—the '*jet*'—becoming project, *projet*.
And I ask the image takers:
– 'What is your project?'
They hesitate, and each has their own way of hesitating. They say:
– 'To make a film . . . '
And we are entirely in agreement.

– 'To make a film—to what end?'
– 'To resist the invader . . . ?'

We are entirely in agreement.
As soon as an arm is in need of a certain number of servants, the human spider will weave—unbeknownst to everyone—and between no less than the crew members of a bomber carrying napalm, phosphorus, and whatever else comes to mind: *porteur, transporteur, projeteur*—a carrier, transporter, projector. When it comes to what people do, the spider couldn't care less.

The human exists on board a tank, as long as there are three or four people inside it; there exists more 'human' still at the target itself, as long as there are some people there waiting. The human exists everywhere—there is a profusion of human; it sprouts up like a weed.

And what I say to the image takers is that weeds have a bad reputation: they're harmful to cultures, and we can say that in a way, cultures are in fact harmful to weeds.

Human being has no need whatsoever for cinema; yet cinema exists, on the basis of which screens small and big are invaded. We need to resist, to give up a small corner of the skylight, gain a notch through which one sees images that strike, and that strike because, quite simply, they're images, and not as a result of what's seen (by the self), for it's here that the paradox lies; the human is not seen (by the *self*); if the human is present, cinema can't help but entail certain stirrings, be in tune, and in harmony. Thus appear images.

But then the image taker must be human himself. . . .
I very much fear that a comment such as this literally means nothing, and that the person who believes they comprehend it, who acknowledges it, the person who, in sum, accepts it, in truth runs a great risk of wanting to convey something; and in considering themself more human than those similar to them, their fellow beings, this person will believe they have the right and the duty to project themself, that they're exemplary. *One* doesn't give a royal damn, as everyone, being *le roi de son soi*—the king of oneself—is a subject.

This I say to the image takers so they're on guard against a certain obviousness that would make necessary a certain degree of connivance between themselves and the *one* who sees the film.

This connivance seems to impose itself because the person who makes the film and the one who sees it are similar. Now, images are coincidence and not at all connivance.

If the person who makes the film looks for connivance, they'll find it easily—to the detriment of the coincidences that are in fact the weeds of the undertaking, since willing them to occur is useless; the image taker can do nothing other than respect them in passing, even though they are not seen: they are undertones, are underviewed, underperceived.

4 - The word similar, which is so simple, should cause image takers to be on guard.

Instead of talking about the screen, I'll talk to them about the wall; fossils have a hard life and the act of tracing on a wall goes back a long time.
Fossils have a hard life.
Every stone is worth taking, even if it becomes necessary to throw it.
All that a trace on the wall awaits, in order to be made—*se faire*—is a hand that finds itself at work, so to speak.
A trace awaits being made—*se faire*; a trace awaits to make this—*ce faire*. . . .Everything made—*tout faire*—then, is a fossil.
Where does the bison etched in the wall come from? From the wall first; there remains the déjà vu . . . The *prévu*, so to speak—what is foreseen. And this is what I say to the image takers, that images, like all that which is alive, are prone to being reproduced.

The image takers have already been to the cinema, and regardless of their intentions, images are prone to being reproduced; there is nothing the image takers can do about this, or nearly nothing, except understand, once and for all, that it's the case, and thus say to themselves, once and for all, that pretentions of originality are completely preposterous. Incidentally, they'll need to realise that words ending in 'ity' are the fiercest enemies of those images that are not part of this world; what is termed 'personality' entails a sense of belonging to a certain world taken to an extreme, and if image takers are going to be part of a guild of sorts, it might as well be one whose members are a bit silly looking and don't have much to say, just as I often see painters or sculptors who are awkward, gawky, when they gesture about their work.

In attempting to be an image taker, one has good reason to be bewildered, especially if it's understood that images are not seen (by the self). If images really truly are not seen (by the self), loquacity—deprived of its support and its raison d'être, which is all that which concerns the *self*—wilts and fades. But where then are the images?

As someone who does nothing but relate and narrate, my gospel is a book—every faith needs one. It's by a good savant who happens to be deaf, which we see in his photo: there's a small string coming out of his ear, and he's all smiles and even full of laughter; who knows what's making this man laugh, since he's clearly as deaf as can be. No doubt what he's looking at. Now, what he's looking at can be seen in a photo on the cover: a tiger spider spinning its web.

And this is what I say to the image takers, without mentioning the spider: Who knows where among the termites the project resides—that of building nests that are architecturally astonishing. The spiders have found something better to ventilate their galleries than that which bees rely on—namely, the flapping of their wings; air passes and circulates through the galleries before which our engineers, who are specialists in ventilation, are dumbfounded.

That said, where would the project be located in a colony containing tens of millions of individuals? There, where the images are located. One can see that *there* is particularly rich where the termite mound, the beaver dam, the badger burrow, or anything else that comes to mind, is thriving, and this includes the spider's web, and the migration of sparrows, and—how about that—even the semi-rigid skeletons of certain organisms that insist on making all their parts themselves, as they have always done and no doubt will continue to do, forever or nearly so.

The Man—that we are—imagines things; on the basis of which, some people—and there are plenty of them—think that the things we all imagine can be seen in projected images.

A completely preposterous idea, but one that undoubtedly reigns; it's a conviction. Yesterday, an image taker told me that when he and I talked, as we were doing; when we conversed; he was driven by morals. He hesitated on the word. At the time, the word he needed didn't come to me; it deals with a practice, a practice that—if it's not to remain weak and even flimsy—must reinforce itself with rigour; as one says that cement is as reinforced as it can be.
And he told me about a minor event that occurred quite recently; while he was grappling with the project of making a film, what was said between us brought about a reshuffling of the usual minor constellation of habits and customs in cinema.
I should have told him that he hadn't seen the end of this, if he had begun to believe what was said between us; one of these days, the camera would end up being the obstacle. While I was making a film, we placed the camera on its three legs, and it gave me stitches—I'm not sure where, but it was like when someone says they have stitches in their side—and so the real find was to hang the camera from the end of a long rod similar to that the Chinese used to transport luggage; for a shoulder, we used

the gimbal of a truck that had been found at a scrap dealer. The fact is that this gimbal was rheumatic, causing jolts in the movements of the camera, which would suddenly jam. A good many of those who saw the film were surprised and it was always during these very moments; the bizarre stops caused, sparked, the image, the image distinctly speaking, and in the very way I mean; that is, an image makes an event, while, quite often, the event that is taken, so to speak, doesn't make an image at all. We have shots of the event and that's about it.

It's easy to comprehend that these stops were due to the rheumatic gimbal and luckily for us, since if the gimbal had not been rheumatic, it would not have been at the scrap dealer. These stops were not seen (by the self)—no more than the counterweight was; at the other end of the rod, it greatly contributed to the strange ease of the camera, an ease that was altogether different from that which would have occurred were the camera held and operated by one of us; a restrained ease.

When it's a matter of a termite mound or an anthill or a village of beavers, lodges, and dams, the image taker must obstinately ask himself where the project is, not in order to respond, but to have an analogy to keep him good company when he asks himself where the images are.

That said, in order for there to be a dam and lodges, there is still need for a river, loose soil, and trees.

This is what I say to the image taker; wherever it is that images are, and come from, the canvas still needs to be there—the river, loose soil, and trees.

I have always been refractory to the word 'screenplay'—to the word and the thing, both of which I'm told are indispensable practices. I don't believe this, and practice by practice, we'll talk about canvas.

The French word for canvas, *canevas*, is old indeed: It was first spotted in 1281, when it was spelled *canevach*, a derivative of *caneva*, which means *chanvre*, or hemp.

At least with hemp, one sees what one's dealing with: a fossil, or nearly so, this *canevach* manufactured from the textile commodity thanks to which one can take off on, or undertake, a sea voyage, to go and inquire if in fact China is not over yonder, China or India or wherever, and then discover America; the hemp from which the cordage is made still needs to resist the assault of the wind in the sails.

We thus have *canevas*: 'Openwork material, light in colour, that serves as the backing for works of needlepoint.'

And this is what I say to the image takers:

– 'The canvas must be coarse and light in colour, and above all, don't forget the holes. If there are no holes, where do you expect the images to land, what do you expect them to come through?'

Is canvas language? It has to be. It would be enough to find a hemp tongue. One has got to exist; language is made of innumerable tongues.

That said, canvas is first of all holes.

Is this to say that I'm going to supply canvases? Lo and behold, the sign for this 'here' that's a regular detour in the image takers' paths would now read: – CANVAS.
And what's the name of the artisan who finds himself in this shop? A canvassor?

To be a fossil to the extent of the being in this shop; he's very much me as I'll never be, and it's too bad. I would have had to live in the Middle Ages; fossils have a hard life; there are numerous fossils in the spirit of the times and that survive if they . . . Hence images, the nostalgia for another era. So much so that a canvassor I am. A canvassor? Someone enters—anyone—and this anyone requests or orders a canvas. If he's a regular customer and he orders a canvas, it will have to be made to order—that is, to his intentions. And so I find myself in the shoes of the cobbler who's concerned for his client's journeys down the road, and the streets his client will take, and for what purpose and with whom; will his client be going to war or out dancing? And what am I meddling in? A canvassor is not really a cobbler; they're completely different.

For some time now, I have been a regular detour in the image takers' paths—whether it be one image taker or the other; their visits are a matter of a practice, or nearly so. And they're a matter of images.

We thus have the canvassor; a strange artisan. Fossils have a hard life. As well as the artisan's shop, there is the odd gallows in the surroundings, Brueghel no doubt having something to do with this; a gallows fossil of sorts.

If you're going to make use of hemp, better do so to make canvas than the hangman's rope.

Canvas; the holes are enclosed by the hemp or it's thanks to the hemp that there are holes.

This is what I say to the image takers as I consider my canvas; it's up to them to take shots in which images appear.

I once knew, and watched from up close, a weaver fossil. He weaved by hand on a large loom; he was a miscreant—in his opinion and in the bottom of his heart; what he wove were ceremonial robes for the monks in an abbey where the stained glass had been made by Matisse.

And I do understand the image taker when he talks to me about painting and music, about how Bach or Beethoven, Braque or Giacometti, would appear in images, if the film he makes has images. I tell him there is no need to worry about the images; it's enough for painting or music to strike them in the right place. It's up to him to prepare the place, so to speak; it's all he can do.

As a canvassor, I would like the canvas to be full of places that are conducive to images.

Cinema is a singular art due to the fact that films don't have authors. But then, as André Bazin said, what about style?

Style no doubt exists, just as images do; one only sees the trace of style and nobody made this trace.
Nobody makes images.
The artisan-weaver certainly didn't have the intention of becoming a priest when he wove the robes; he would have instead thought that as far as priests went, there were already too many.

We don't know what we're doing when it comes to images and we certainly don't know who they'll affect; be that as it may, images are necessary. They're absolutely necessary.

What about chance?
As a canvassor, I can say that all those holes in the hemp's thread open themselves up to chance.

When I talk this way, the two image takers who visit me here—and not together, but one after the other—have very different reactions.

One of them has made chance his close pal; the other doesn't trust it. It's as if he were to say to me:
– 'Chance . . . ? That's just a word.'
Even if he did have this thought, he wouldn't say it. The customary of this network

has its rigours, just like other societies did—those that, truth be told, are fossils they're so archaic. I'm the one who relates, narrates, and philosophises; who's the 'chief', ethnologists of an outdated era would say. It's true that I harp on about stories fossilised and full of truths, and about images, but there are different species of images: there are those born of a hint of story—but are these images, distinctly speaking?—and those traced on a wall.

And the image taker who doesn't seem to believe in chance, or doesn't trust it, tells me that fifteen or more years ago, he found himself with a motley group of four or five other barbarians, one of whom was an American through and through, a marine who had come from Vietnam, after having deserted. They were climbing a small mountain not too far from here, one that is quite steep, in an attempt to reach the ruins of a château said to date back to the Cathars. The marine of repute was the first to arrive; he was an experienced climber and the ascent had been full of perils, as the rock was friable. They had been climbing for hours and had reached the stones of the ruin perched on a peak, when ten metres in front of them, they saw a little old lady with a black straw hat, each hand holding something, one a basket, the other a girl. They were unable to believe their eyes: the old lady proved that ghosts exist—either that or there was a footpath on the other side that climbed gradually to the château.
The question remains whether the climber to arrive first was an authentic marine who had deserted, as the legend of uncertain origin would have it; he himself had not said anything about Vietnam. And who knows if the old lady was not the wife of a Huguenot who had escaped the galleys and hidden in the château's cellar; whether she was on her way to bring him more provisions, accompanied by the little girl who served as a decoy to mislead the priest's spies, or the intendant's, or the dragoon commander's. This is an event fossil that's seen and reiterated in the same form in moment after moment of history, its last appearance dating back to 1943 in this very spot.

What about making a film that entails taking shots of a re-enacted story? It's done; it's even done often.

To the image taker who told me about the event that happened to him fifteen years ago at the Château de F., I say:

– 'You can see that chance exists. . . .You were there by chance. . . .'

He's not at all convinced, and with good reason; he mutters:

– 'In any case, I didn't have a camera; where, pray tell, was I supposed to have put one . . . ?'

And the fact is that chance is not seen (by the self), just as images are not.

Cathars, Camisards, galleys, and gallows—is it a question here of 'naturalising' the ghosts of history?

While I was a communist and in charge of Travail et Culture, not only did I watch films, but I escorted them when they were projected here and there. And in one of these films, Stalin appeared, a naturalised, re-enacted Stalin, played by an actor while Stalin was still very much alive. I have said too much about this event; I have gone on about the Musée Grévin. Have I said too much about it? I have recounted it often, but without getting to the bottom of things, so to speak. The facets of an event are innumerable. If I recounted it in 1969, I offered the visceral anti-Stalinist's facet, even though I was a communist. An event is like a die, a die that has more than six faces. Now, chance is the Arabic word for a die. How about that.

In addition to the face that presented itself when I appeared to be endowed with a quite considerable amount of political intuition, there are thirty others, one of which shows itself today; on seeing the film circulate, I regretted the radical lack of images.

The film was perhaps a matter of imagery that was relevant to the tradition of icons. As for images, there were none.

I came across the proof that fossils have a hard life in a book by César Chavez. It recounts the hard work involved in establishing a union of Chicanos, Mexicans who illegally crossed—and perhaps still do—the Mexican–American border to find jobs in California during the harvest season.[6] In order for the Chicanos to become a bit better organised and resist the bloodsuckers, they had to fight the sheriff and his men, as well as the militia, all of whom were paid by the planters. When there was a worker doing time in jail for some custom-made crime, protestors would gather under the windows of the prison where he was being held. There were two towns nearby, one to the east and one to the west of the site of unrest. When the protest moved towards the prison in the east, there was a crowd of people. When it went west, there were hardly any protestors. For a long time, César Chavez sought an explanation for this surprising phenomenon. And then he found it, and it was certain that in times past, processions followed a route towards the east; procession fossils they thus were, and not ghost processions.

Which images then?
I'm not an image taker.
To naturalise events is to hunt images, track them, eliminate them, place them out of frame from the get go.

How can abuses of power be recognised, whether they be those of a tyrant or those of money? By the massacre of images, their disappearance.

This is why, when I was in charge of Travail et Culture, I grumbled loudly, with the complete innocence of someone protesting—or doing I know not what—anything that took as its project or cause the status accorded the human person. Not that I claim that such a project would be erroneous or fallacious. I don't know anything about that; I chat about images, or rather, about that which could potentially cause images to happen, it being well-understood that images don't cause things to happen[7] any more than birds do, and that they're similar to spiders, which don't squawk and don't have hands and yet spin webs. The image taker doesn't have hands either; they're busy handling the camera, and the camera is not a stone he's going to project like human beings did in times past, when a stone was all it took for them to persist and exist despite everything; and from that stone they threw, a project was born and it expanded as objects diversified and became tools. A tool stranger than the camera? The rigours of the customary mean that I never see that tool.

A canvassor I am and will remain, and from the spider I learnt that while spinning a web, one must always leave a thread without glue; in the same way, I respect the holes that are essential and absolutely necessary if one wants to attempt to obtain images due to chance.

An ant runs across the collimator sight of a machine gun, and in the surroundings, the Spanish Civil War is raging while my mate places a scrap of skin from a priest in his plump wallet, the look on his face as meek as that of a turtle, and an old lady is very much there, atop an inaccessible peak, a black straw hat on her head, a basket in one hand, a girl in the other. She's not a ghost; she herself is not a fossil. She's there, where she is; and *there* or *where* she is, there is human fossil.

If there were images, the old lady could relate her story in the manner of: once upon a time . . .

Once and for all; this entails surprise and finding again.

Images are not finds but what is found again.

This is what I harp on about to the image takers:

– 'Along with what can be seen, there is seeing, and the vacancy of making seeing out to be seeing again. . . .'

For those who have not lived close to 'autistic' beings, what I say falls into the void, so to speak. Not an ounce of understanding to be expected.

That said, autistic beings are of the human species; alas, they're only human; put otherwise, they're not 'they', since the 'they' they're assumed to be doesn't take, has not found a means of taking hold, has not come across something to take hold of; which happens throughout nature, to innumerable seeds.

Nevertheless, they have taught me that *voir*, to see, is *revoir*, to see again, the 're' in French being due to a kind of memory—one that belongs to the same species as that which reminds the beaver how to make its dam so that it turns out a dam.

And what's surprising about the fact that human being is endowed with this memory? The opposite would be surprising.
That said, the Man that we are has an image of himself, as it were, and this image is not, distinctly speaking, an image, but imagery, the product of naturalisation; Man is his own icon—the icon is incorporated.

The image taker then—but why 'taker'? One should say charmer—exorcise the icon and there you go. And I'm not talking about devils emerging; I'm talking about images, because where do images emerge from? From whoever sees them, and this seeing is seeing again; but who has already seen what will be seen again? No person; no subject, at any rate.

The image taker is a bit stunned and with good reason, I admit. No person sees these images—in person—and no person takes them.

– 'That's it exactly . . . ' says the canvassor and gets back to work, the work being made of hemp and vacancy, and the vacancy not being taken by the hemp; on the contrary, the hemp is what makes it possible.

And look at the coincidence: in around 1280, *canevas* was referred to as *canevach* in French—*vach* like in *vaguer*, to wander, and not *vacher*, a cowherd.

5 - I used to have, I had, another mate; he was called Poirier, and he was endowed, by nature, with a certain richness in attitude fossils.
We were soldiers together: same year, same season, same citadel barracks; Vauban having something to do with this.

He was unable to stretch his arms out completely, like a gorilla or a Japanese wrestler or whatever comes to mind that trudges along and moves towards you, arms half bent and dangling, the elbow joint inadvertently stuck.
Canvas; I'll tell the image takers about this: In the vacant hole, chance had the regimental band enter the barracks courtyard to play 'La Marseillaise' for us, and Poirier began to jump about, to gambol; he danced the jig or the mazurka. If I tell the image takers about this, where will they go to take shots of an event like it, one that is truly remarkable? It's too late; the event dates back to 1936.

But what I want to say to the image takers is that they have to keep an eye out; an event such as this could always happen.

– 'Why not,' one of them says to me, while the other, shaking his head, thinks he'd have to be damn lucky.

What I say in response is that an event like this is very much a fossil; at all times, in all places, on all occasions, there is a Poirier who begins to gambol out of moment, and so it depends: He may be hung or applauded, pilloried or glorified as though he were king; he may become mottled with blows or stuffed full of intentions. What remains is the image that each of us forms in the imagery of our liking, which occurs when we tell ourselves what the image represents and means.

As far as I'm concerned, the fact is that images don't represent anything at all. That's why they're images; they themselves have no signification.

Anyone who says sign, says code; you might as well tell wild geese to respect the Highway Code or the Air Traffic Code.

Now, whether he likes it or not, the image taker lives in connivance with his fellow beings; as such, he either pleases them or defies them. In both cases, his message is coded, so to speak. Has one ever seen a message that was not coded? One would not comprehend any of it; or 'see' any of it.

To say that images have meaning and that they're carriers of messages makes me think of pigeons that have a small band around their leg or in their feathers; the band is a message and the pigeons are in charge of it.

But the image taker is saddened by this. If he listens to me, does he have to make a film that doesn't mean anything?

The canvassor would never, ever say such a thing.
That which doesn't mean anything refers to a large group of run-of-the-mill pretentions,

while when I talk about cinema, I'm talking about a popular art, the popular being quite fond of simply comprehending what one wishes—to mean—even if doing so entails the perception of images when they appear. This is what stirrings entail.

I'll have to distinguish between being stirred and experiencing emotion. Over time, words go limp, get mixed up. People borrow them and stick them any old place.

Talking about *émoi* has removed the content from the word, just as one does the escargot from its shell. Stirrings? One is stirred and for no reason at all; stirrings are not seen and one doesn't question the causes or the reason.

Do they exist? Images exist. Images are not seen (by the self). They are traces. Are traces seen? Certain traces are seen (by the self) and others are not. Those that are not seen are thus lost, erased; it's useless to talk about them.

Which is precisely why these traces need to be talked about, even if only to say that doing so erases them. To perceive them, one would need a third eye. This third eye exists, even if only in Tibet; it exists there in the customs and habits of thought of the bonzes, some of whom go so far as to pierce it between their other two eyes, mid-forehead. And what do they see then? Who knows . . .
The image takers are in agreement when I say to them that, all things considered, the camera's a better bet. They're ready for everything except perhaps putting a hole in their frontal wall. That said, even if it's only because of their habit of viewing what the camera has taken, the range of their gaze is altered: now look what regards them.

A canvassor, I return to my *métier*.[8]
While I peaceably weave the canvas being made, I don't foresee the embroidery. The adorned is the image taker's to-do.[9] For fifteen years, we have lived close to autistic children, and between us, we have used jargon for our métier, assuming that living close is a métier.

Canvassing is a métier; to put it better, in order to canvas, a *métier*, a loom, is needed—a small loom, one quite a bit smaller than the weaving loom used by the artisan whose house shook from top to bottom by the impact of its reed, which was released by a cord, the movement made being the same as that of the blacksmith-farrier who worked a bellows to fan embers.

Mine is about forty by thirty centimetres, the format of the sheet of paper on which I write of canvases full of holes. The tapestry will be adorned—when the film is made.

Between us, we know what the adorned is all about: the reiterated detours that are the gestures of being when talking doesn't intervene—neither talking, nor saying to oneself—and that occur in the vacancy of the project to be carried out.

As far as I'm concerned, adorning is human. Which is where the fossil reappears, and between us, the use of the maps that unled us astray while we were first learning about the existence areas.
At the same time, there we were, grappling with the shooting areas.
What does foreseeing entail? There, where the camera is placed, such that here and there, and as though on a detour in the foreseen paths of those who will be in the frame, a blossom of small circles appears, and we trace it with the same gesture we used to encircle the binding joists, a word in our jargon that designates the very specific places where the autistic beings' paths cross via the moments that make up the days, weeks, months, and years, and via the individuals who are autistic beings.

And these binding joists are very much proof of the existence of traces that are not seen, because the traces really do have to exist in order for the kids, male or female, to get their bearings relative to the binding joists, after years of distance and whether or not they're with their close presences.

Finding the right place to put the camera is not inscribed in the canvas. It's the work of the image taker; just the same, the old canvassor that I am has got to ramble on, even if only in honour of the image takers who visit him, as he's a regular detour in their paths.

Adorning is human and in a primordial way, just as throwing and tracing are human, and one can clearly see the difference between adorning, which is acting, and doing or making anything, including a film.

Adorning—what could be more natural? One need only look to innumerable animal species. Humans thus appear quite defenceless, though they do have hands, and so one need only look to their skin, *la peau*, and their rags, *les oripeaux*, and then, on the wall . . .

On the wall, the screen, one sees what's projected and wonders what it represents, and what it means, on a detour in the course of daily or weekly life.

And it's there that the war rages, and not the war of images, but guerrilla warfare—in order for there to be images.

What's the use in talking about totalitarian regimes? All of cinema circulates formidable imagery. As soon as images appear, there are stirrings; the return of the storks and no need to see the bird. Images come back . . .

This is why I canvas and ramble on.
I have a long-standing habit of useless breaches. The adorned is not useful though it is necessary and perhaps indispensable. Fossils have a hard life but species occasionally disappear.

The human being disappears and people don't feel anything is absent. People have a long-standing habit of rendering the human being nearly or entirely absent. We're in the *nearly*, it seems to me, which is not at all surprising if one considers that the human being doesn't make signs.

When it comes to communication between individuals of the same species, there is not a single animal species that has lessons to learn from humans. Having said that, humans discovered the sign and they seem to believe it's sufficient; the sign is where the human disappears, gradually becoming a fossil. Is every fossil a trace? Traces are not made and they don't make signs—traces don't make signs; neither do images. Attitudes can make signs. Music doesn't make signs, hence opera, though it's not the music that's talking: it's Wagner, or Mozart when he feels like it, Mozart or the librettist, and behind them, the Freemasonry, and this is just fine.

I had a teacher; he was a freemason. We had no idea. The Nazis did. They didn't misfire. When he arrived at the school's courtyard, he would remain standing, take a watch from his pocket, and swing it by the chain. While he did this, he didn't make any signs. An adorned gesture. Such is the image that I see again. He talked a lot and well; he was a remarkable teacher. The image that returns to me doesn't say anything and in fact is not an image of him—in person, I mean. A human gesture; and some people are richer than others in gestures of this nature; they're clowns, and one knows to what extent they're fossils.

Hemp is vacant, it's the canvas.
And lo and behold, I foresee images in the vacancy, and it's not that I see the images but that I believe we can expect chance, the adorned. . . .

The holes are full; they're overflowing.
Not at all. Chance, the adorned, images—all come from the same hemisphere and of the three, only the adorned takes up space; chance can't be captured; images do nothing other than pass by; they're always in migration.

The adorned is not made of signs, regardless of what one says. Signs need somewhere to land—why not on the adorned?

Having said this, I relate and narrate a minor event that took place in the asylum where I lived for five years—so the image takers might glimpse what the adorned entails.

Every year, during the same time of year, there were kids who escaped. Suffice it to say that the escape occurred right before springtime and that the kids, big or small, sensed the lure of whatever might come to mind. Escaping was not easy. A good deal of planning was needed and everything had to be foreseen and planned without the kids being spotted.

And what I emphasise to the image takers is that the small band of five or seven that would form was a motley group of individuals.

Some of the individuals could have been regarded as intelligent and recidivists; but what about the others? If the leaders were intelligent, why did they coagulate with the kooks who were obviously stupid, hindrances, inept?

Why they did eludes us and we won't speak of it further; one is well aware that in an instant, a film concerned with *why* drains itself of any of the attraction it might have. There remains *how*. How did these five or seven kids find themselves in a group planning their escape? This is what I say to the image takers: If you manage to film *how*, people will establish relationships—but the word is hackneyed—connections, whatever comes to mind, with one another, and as a result they'll get each other's goat; if one is willing to agree that for the goat, the flock entails unity, then the image takers will have learnt their métier. One might say that the kids sent each other signs; the sign takes the blame, and I have nothing against the sign except that it hinders and hides what one should attempt to grasp in passing—in the moment of its passing; the rest, all the rest, is a potential informer. The band, the flock, that formed was a fossil; it was human like in times past, an out-of-sign human; I would bet my life on it, I who witnessed it first-hand.[10]

One might talk to me about projects; the word is ludicrous, and not the word but the object of the project, which is not in fact the end.

Canvas; locked up in an asylum—an asylum or a prison or a penitentiary, it doesn't matter which—some individuals among a hundred others plot their escape together. Now, escaping is not the end; it's the pretext, the necessary decoy so that a band of five or seven can plot together—in order for doing so to be proposed, imposed, and become the project, because it's there that the only possible project lies. There are no others within reach. And so to camer what this could be and what eludes understanding. Images might appear.

And such is the case with every canvas: hemp and holes, vacant air, and then chance.

Does the image taker abhor chance? If it's not him who does, it's the producer, hence the screenplay and the strange habits of cinema that prove the extent to which the fossil has a hard life; sometimes, it would seem, images appear below the surface. And what's the use in talking about cinema?

Do the image taker and canvassor thus form a pair? Perhaps; this is what I have been telling myself these days, and in telling it to myself, I tell it to the both of us. And we have gotten on well each of these days; we have been in a harness together.
I want to say that images do nothing other than appear on the screen and to say that the slightest of shots taken requires tedious, intense work; this remark appears to be contradictory, paradoxical. The image takers are full of paradoxes. All that I relate and ramble on about is peppered with them, which seems to me the best way for the image takers to have a free hand. They have a choice: they can either be bewildered, and with good reason, or leave me where I am, a regular detour: departure and return, or at the very least passing through, and when they visit me here, the image takers don't have a camera slung over their shoulders.

It would appear that there are those who take the screen for a dustbin. When a product is shown on one, what's seen is what's found in dustbins: packaging. Having said this, it doesn't concern me.

Don't forget that the use of the camera makes it possible to see a plant grow—a few months in only a minute.

It's quite certain that when a person discovers something they rarely think of the chain reaction that their finding will bring about.

The inventor of the camera discovered what was to become a funfair attraction, or nearly one, and then lo and behold, there were image takers with debonair looks and a certain mastery of time and space.

What takes place on the screen, which is on the wall, ricochets there, having come from anywhere, and time subjects the necessary commotion to attraction. We're there without being there and we're used to it.

Attraction? The dictionary gives us: – that which attracts the public – force that attracts (law of universal gravitation).

And this is what I say to the image takers: as filmmakers, you create an attraction.

Which is where the two gravities reappear—the ones that put me at a great risk of being taken for a kook.

Everyone experiences the attraction of universal gravitation, and in daily life, no one thinks about it; that it's there is a fact, so much so that it doesn't need us to exist, to occur. And then, lo and behold, on top of this attraction—which one can say one is unaware of, though this unawareness clearly differs from that which is talked about, and language certainly has something to do with this—along comes the attraction of what takes place on the wall, and it snatches folks away from the drudgery of existence.

Periods of commotion are part of existence for mankind, and these periods are fossils, or to put it better, fossil lies below their surface. The protest of unionised Chicanos readily follows the inclination of past processions and there have always been detours in the course of vernacular routes, side trips often taken because they held some attraction, gravity prevailing for a moment over the urgent need to do what had to be done.

Vernacular? The word may surprise.
It speaks to us of that which is distinct to a country, and below the word's surface is: – verna, a slave born in the household. Thus appears the slave, and it can be said that, when it comes to TV, plenty of folks of all ages are slaves.

Since words allow something entirely different than what's understood to appear below the surface, look what appears when we examine this word a little more closely: – prehension. It entails *prehendere*, which means: action of grasping, of taking; faculty of grasping with an appropriate organ.

I write while the image takers are not here.

I await their visit so I can tell them that as image takers, they have an appropriate organ, one that enables the prehension of images.

Now, lo and behold, from the word prehension arise appendices: comprehension and apprehension—huge words; insatiable monsters. Comprehension and apprehension are very attractive; the everyperson wants to comprehend, and delights in apprehending, all the more so because what happens doesn't happen to them. The first misfortune that befell cinematography, when it was a funfair attraction, was that the room emptied before the train that was arriving, the everyperson believing that the train arriving at the station was coming straight at them. We're no longer there. Anything can happen on the wall and the worse it is, the more the every-person rejoices intimately that it's happening without happening to them—or else what happens is they feel as though they were there, or nearly so; it depends.

Nearly . . . The image taker is equipped with an organ thanks to which he will be projected from *nearly*. Nearly is almost nothing, is almost *as though*.

The fact remains that between comprehension and apprehension, the distance is considerable.

In times past, apprehension meant comprehension; the two words, still close to their origin, coincided, and then they separated and apprehension came to mean: – operation by which the spirit attains a simple object of thought, as opposed to comprehension, which assumes a complex object. And then, much later, fear appeared, a vague fear, poorly defined, alarm, anguish, anxiety, worry, fear, foreboding.

And this is quite often one of the filmmaker's artifices: We anticipate what is going to happen, we see it coming—either that, or we don't expect it. In any case, this is not the moment to bewilder us with art and artifice. It's the organ that I foresee discussing with the image takers. An organ, how about that . . .
It's not very surprising that human beings have organs that grow, among them, language, which followed tools, and then with the help of language, tools were perfected and diversified, and what happened is that these organs came to exist to the detriment of human beings, even though they seemed to be to their advantage.

It's an old story, entirely fossilised, that of a species in which certain organs or certain adornments become profuse and then the species disappears as a result of profusion.

As a result of a profusion of equipment, the hand will atrophy; but the person who says 'hand' speaks of hemispheres, and more specifically, that hemisphere on which the apprehension of distance depends.

The baboon apprehends the branch it will grab hold of.

Just as the human being, stone in hand, apprehends the reach of their throw.

And lo and behold, along comes an organ that puts everything and anything within everyone's reach, within reach, or nearly so.

Anything that can take place on the screen doesn't concern me.

That said, apprehending works, and as soon as seeing, as it were, and even before—as soon as hearing, as soon as being.

This is a fact.

A canvassor I am, and being one entails the canvas; the rambling is just so I'm good company in the presence of the image takers.

One can clearly see how many falsifications could occur, and have occurred, as a result of profusion, ever since the appearance of the *instrument* that enables us to see, in an instant, a plant growing, and enables us to be there, wherever that may be, to be there, or nearly so.

Once upon a time there were artisan weavers who discovered an artifice that allowed them to see the threads of a fabric, the warp and the weft, from up close, this artifice being a piece of curved glass: the magnifying glass. And then, lo and behold, came the microscope and all that followed, and then the movie camera after the still camera, and the telescope to see stars or ships.

As artisans, what do the image takers make? They make *nearly*, and so it's like being in a well-stocked cheese shop; when it comes to nearly, there is something for every taste, hundreds of varieties, or rather breeds, of nearly, and if not breeds, then brands. There are those that are nearly authentic and those given the designation of origin, those from Holland, from Cantal or Auvergne, and the nearly nearly, nearly pâté, nearly preserve, cooked nearly, adulterated nearly. The same goes for what comes out of the instrument that is a newcomer and already well incorporated, even if only in habits and customs.
Has it been mastered? Here we are.
If one is something of a slave to the screen—small or big—who's the master?
The next time I see the image takers in turn, I'll say:
– 'What's the compass used for . . . ?'
Response:
– 'To find your way . . . to see.'

I'll say:

– 'To realise there are poles. And so then what's the instrument called a camera used for? To detect the existence—time and again—of the human being and the fact that the human being's attractiveness exerts itself without our knowledge.'

If cinema is an attraction—which it is—one sees the role and necessity of this attraction. Images feel the effects of, are derived from, the attractiveness of the human being.

And here we are: shots taken and, in this prehension, there is the apprehension of the human being.

Is this to say that we're going to become, go towards, the human being . . . ? The fact that there are poles—which the compass displays, demonstrates—doesn't mean every navigator goes towards them; that would be migration and disaster. The Man—that we are—already has enough whims and it would not be opportune to add another.

There is human being in the *nearly*; there is, or rather, there could—perhaps—be, even if only an ounce.

An ounce of human being in the *nearly* and the image takers will be able to tell themselves that they have not lived in vain.

That said, the task is a difficult one. They will need tenacity, dexterity, moderation, humility, genius, and whatever else comes to mind that is ceaselessly squandered throughout the world.

As a canvassor, I do what I can.
When the image takers visit me here, they leave their instrument of choice at home, as 'here' is not their home; it's no more, no less, than an inn that's a regular detour in their paths.

Fossils have a hard life; there exist innumerable inns, guesthouses, pensions—or whatever else comes to mind—and there are quite a few folks who believe it's necessary to add an attraction on top of what makes the place attractive, even though its attractiveness lies in the fact that it's en route. Nevertheless, the everyperson will ask themself: Why go? And so now they can say it's because of the attraction, which has been thrown into the bargain, so to speak. The attraction is just a matter of conscience; good or bad, it matters little.

Once upon a time the owners of cinemas chose the films that appeared on their screens; a bygone era. There is distribution, which determines awards, and awards, which determine the distribution of whatever comes to mind where the institution is profuse.

But this in fact doesn't concern me. I'm not even capable of creating a non-profit organisation, I'm unfit.

However, I am a canvassor—by instinct, so to speak—just as Mr Laurens was a sculptor all along, according to his son.

A canvassor to such an extent that for years, I happened to live equipped with that instrument called a camera, which was there because I managed to procure one for myself. Though apparently, for want of funds, there was no film.

And what happened then? And then everything happened as if there was one, the everyperson who took part in the fortnight living and acting, at all times, as though the film had arrived from god knows where, just like manna in the desert.

And the fact is that a downward drift was entirely perceptible, a drift compared to what the every-person would have been if . . . If the camera had not been there.
Is this to say that the every-person thus played a role? The every-person always plays a role, camera or no camera; the role became entirely different—even though I hadn't given, cast, assigned roles.

A canvassor I am, and nothing else, and all along, and when it comes to my métier, no one taught it to me, not my father, nor my grandfather. It's innate. It's a gift. Everybody has one, and I made a métier, or nearly did, of mine. A common gift, certainly, and I say so to the image takers; the human being is a canvassor; this is clear to me, but if they want to go and take a look near, and around, folks who don't suspect it to be the case, they'll need the instrument that's endowed with a certain capacity for prehension—and the instrument won't be sufficient. They'll still need a wall, and on the wall, a screen. To look at a screen that is empty, white, ivory, or greyish makes me think of that scrap of skin that was square, or nearly so, and about the size of the palm of one's hand—the priest's skin. And the priest was not seen on the scrap, not the priest, nor the tree, nor the well, nor the rifle, nor the target aimed at the lad in the Brigades with his barrel or jerrycan, nor the Spanish Civil War.

And this screen, on the wall—what is it the skin of? And if not skin, *peau*, then *oripeau*, frill; the screen, *lambeau d'oripeau*, a scrap of frill; should a painter stop by and canvas be lacking, he'll get down to it, and it's not that he'll get down to it *on* and *in* the screen, but that his hands will get to work. Or else what will appear? A quartermaster, from back when there were schooners; he'll be in quest of the section of his topgallant sail that was cut a mere two hundred years ago, and since that day, he'll have been searching, not for a ghost, but for a fossil.

What is one searching for? You've got to figure that all the folks who go look at the screen are missing something, since the screen holds an attraction for them. Who knows what *one* might be missing, what *one* is deprived of. What is *one* missing? Nothing.

'To apprehend' is an infinitive; put otherwise, it's insatiable.

It's enough for there to be a hole in a wall, one no bigger than a screen, for human being to go and see. See what? Nothing. See. That said, human being is not the only species there; go ask the rats what they see, or the crows, or anything else that takes a good look, picks up on a scent, apprehends.

That said, every species has its way of apprehending.

It's quite simple; the beaver apprehends, and if by apprehending—which could be called investigating—it discovers a river, loose soil, trees, it won't be long before the dam and lodges occur by themselves. 'Selves'? Who knows . . .

This is what I say to the image takers; the human is always on the point of occurring by *itself*; all that is missing are the indices and indices are not signs, though the dictionary says they are; even if it means uprooting the word so that *indice*, index, makes me think instead of *indicible*, inexpressible.

Investigate? The French verb for 'investigate', *investiguer*, doesn't exist in the dictionary of words in use.[11] 'Investigation', *investigation*, and 'investigator', *investigateur* are there; *investiguer* is not; a remarkable absence; when an infinitive is evasive, there is a strong possibility that the person will go after it, eliminate it.

Is the human always on the point of occurring by *itself*? Like the beaver lodge? More so like world peace, which in the process of occurring by *itself* doesn't occur, never occurs, doesn't succeed in occurring.

Here one sees that willing something to happen is not sufficient, neither is wishing for it to occur, nor is anything that is thought or said (by the *self*).

Canvas: a big fellow who's a bit backwards—*demeuré*—wanders around the cellar into which his companion has disappeared and clearly won't be able to get *himself* out of.

The big fellow returns from the river where he has filled a can of preserves with water.

On his way back up, he confuses one house—*demeure*—with another. On the ceiling, he sees the sun's light reflected off the water in the can. He watches; he sits down. What could be more human?

What could be more human than to watch a reflection flicker on the ceiling? In doing this, he's not human; his companion has been stuck in the cellar for days; the cellar has become a vault.

As for the companion, we no longer hear him. So the big fellow proceeds to his burial; he piles up stones and prays, his hands together, a priest and a congregant at the same time. What could be more human? It's said, in ethnological parlance, that the cult of the dead marks the difference between people and animals.

The big backwards fellow is decidedly not human—or is he too human?

Human? There has been an abuse of the word; the word abuses us.

Investiguer, then, since there is no verb form. If the word is not there, the thing could exist.

To be—in the infinitive—in the human mode is to be unaware of the cadastre. Individuals of this species exist somewhere, in a small group of around thirty. Someone arrives from the savanna or the forest or the river—it matters little. Will they be welcomed, or knocked out? That depends; it's entirely uncertain.

One understands nothing about the human in being.
And now the latest news is that a Syrian cineaste, a naturalised American, has just made a million-dollar film that recounts, in the Libyan desert, the Arabs' fight against the Italians when the state was fascist.[12] Ten thousand extras and the re-enactment, with tanks and cannons, of a period that is still very recent, very much smouldering, or nearly so. As for smoke, there's some in Beirut, the director would have thought; a quick shot of the—authentic—smoke rising from the rubble in Beirut and then, through editing, one will see the Libyan desert smouldering. One assumes one will be content indeed. The screen will be occupied for one hundred and fifty minutes.
The story will easily tell and edit *itself*.

As for being—in the infinitive—that's another kettle of fish, and another métier altogether, even though the instrument is the same; at times the camera is an instrument and at times it's an organ; it depends.

6 - In reality, and to be completely honest, I made the canvas I just described while writing; the film has existed for nearly twenty years.

I was there, the chief of artillery, at the camera: three years of shooting, and prior to that, ten years of living as a close presence to the character, the big backwards fellow.

'Collimator' exists in the dictionary, as does 'collimation'. *Collimater*, 'to collimate', is missing.

The infinitives have deserted, and at the same time, as it were: *investiguer*, *collimater*.

We'll borrow 'to apprehend' then, and what I have in fact apprehended is to place my eye where I should. Chief of artillery or not, project manager, or whatever else, when it comes to the rear sight, I won't give it a glance.
A canvassor I am, and nothing else, even if it means spending years preparing a canvas that may or may not turn out to be a canvas. Let's just say that I cultivate hemp, that I even spin it, but why do it? I really don't know. Time will tell.
The image takers arrive, they're fossils; they could be knife grinders, tinkers mending earthenware and china, traders dealing in bric-a-brac, or anyone who asks if there are images to be taken.

I'm a canvassor, but this is not seen; on seeing me, you would think I was a writor, and if the pages written by this writor are published, here he is, the writer.

Some know I'm a writer; they arrived this way; they have read me. The image takers would do well to make a film. . . .

Here I am, a canvassor, which works out better for me than writing from where I write—what I recount will never be popular. Now, what's popular counts, and it exists.

The human in being will remain a fossil until the day that what's popular . . .

In this regard, as in many others, the image takers and I are as one. If a film makes *itself*, who knows what the *self* doing the making is.

To apprehend, then . . . ?
The dictionary informs us: *saisir au corps*, to catch and arrest . . .
Où est le corps, where is the body that has been arrested? It has to be identified. What does? If it can't be identified, one can try to find analogies. . . . This is what I do when I ramble on.
I say:

– 'If images are something, this something takes after the bird, the bird and the spider, and if not the spider, the beaver; creation is not sufficient. It's possible that the human has never been created; the creator wanted to see; he created all the species, and on arriving at the human, said to himself: – These birds will manage on their own; they'll invent themselves, they'll find their own clockwork.'

There you have it: what the great clockmaker no doubt thought. Because it's very much the case that the beaver's projects—its dam and lodge—are well incorporated; same goes for the spider and its web, and the migration of sparrows and geese, and the termite and its mound, and whatever else comes to mind that is very much fixed.

Reste l'humain, en plan. The human remains, stranded. And when this happens, there is not even a plan. One comprehends nothing of it.

This is what I say to the image takers. There is no plan. The creator has forgotten—as far as we're concerned—to write the screenplay. If there had been a commission with an advance on earnings, we would not have happened, we would not have been welcomed. This project must be redone, the president would have said; worst case scenario, we can vote for a writing assistant, to write a screenplay, one that's done correctly. The story is full of holes. Of course it is; it's a canvas; it's not a story.

– 'The human is not the lodge—the lodge of life. The human is a point, a pole.'

I happened to see a camera with the photocell incorporated. And I said so to the image takers; I said to them:

– 'What is it that you need? There's a compass . . . When you look through the sights and move towards true images, you'll see the needle . . . '

And that's how the man who taught me certain rudiments of elementary philosophy, no more than a few vocabulary words, got taken away by the Nazis. He took his watch for a compass. Time? He was of another time. A fossil and old-fashioned to the extent that a clown can be.

These comments that I harp on about, rehash, they're like quid—just a little something to tinge my ramblings.

I'm determined to make canvases, and come to think of it, one might believe they're in a frame-maker's shop—imagine that. Or if not in a frame-maker's shop, an artisan's, one who makes frames, frames like there's no tomorrow, while waiting for a spider to apprehend them . . . spiders? Imagine that. Who knows where the spiders will make their web—on the ceiling, in the corners of windows.

And what happens is that an image taker comes by to tell me that he has seen a web. So I say to him:

– 'You'll have to bring it to me . . . I'll frame it . . . put it in a canvas . . . put a canvas all around it. . . .'

The image taker would like nothing better, even if only to please me, but there's no chance. . . .The spider's web can't be transported just like that; it's a lot harder to capture than a butterfly; wherever it is, it takes hold. One has got to see a spider at work. I tell the image takers this because there are plenty of lessons to be learnt. The spider situates itself on a branch and makes you an ultra-thin thread that continues to elongate, the spider having placed—in its manner—glue on the free end, a tiny bit of glue. The spider chose this branch because it was in the wind, and would have apprehended that there was something around to work with—another branch or the corner of a wall for the thread to stick to. If the thread sticks, that's it, the spider is good to go. . . .

As for myself, I'm making a canvas, and the image taker crouches down—morally—where he likes, then lets go of the thread; all that's needed is wind. And the image taker says to me:

– 'The thread is fine; it's the glue that I can't get right. . . .'

Well now . . . is finding the glue the work of the canvassor? Or is the image taker talking about glue because he has lost the thread and doesn't want to appear . . .

It's easy to comprehend that if the image taker and the canvassor quarrel, it's all over; it's a fragile thing, the spider's web, it's precarious; one word too many and you realise that words are worse than bumblebees; than Maybugs.

Twenty years have passed, and as a writor, I regret the canvas of that film for which I was project manager; what a mess . . . Ten hours of film exposed and then what? A few images, perhaps . . . At least there were a few: the clumsy hands that are not able to tie a knot and then these hands becoming something other than hands, something that swirls and spins, caught in the whirlwinds and eddies of chance, and I'm well aware of what happens to them, to these hands; they try to make like, and to make like what's happening is that they're managing it, but it's by *making like* that the knot isn't tied, doesn't tie itself, which doesn't happen to the beaver's lodge or dam; the beaver doesn't *make like*—not like its father or its mother or its grandfather or any other beaver it would have seen make a lodge or dam.

There is no other for the beaver.
And as for the human, do I mean being in the mode of a singular species that considers itself humane? It's true, of course, that the other exists, but like humans, beavers live quite harmoniously in small groups. The fact is that they don't give a damn about making like the other, whoever that may be.

For the image taker, it's possible that apprehending entails the thread of what could be if the other had neither place nor course to follow.

What a surprise and what a relief; how evident, also; thus appear images, detectable by the stirrings they bring about; the one-every is only forsaken if they're there—if one is not there, and thus neither is the other, what happens, what thread unfolds?

Because the sign, which some people believe is, marks, the difference between people and animals, requires—in order to occur and enable singular communication between one person and another—that what unites one and the other be entrenched; then, lo and behold, this one and this other are created. There is a code, and thus a detour, that must be apprehended—a detour that is inevitable and that becomes all the more pressing, and constraining, because the reigning doctrines multiply the objurgations that become an exorcism.

I have long wondered what these recommendations and pre-emptory advice aim to exorcise; to name, one has no choice but to name, to name immediately, and at every opportunity—in order to exorcise what? Silence? I had this thought and at the same time found the idea preposterous: How could silence be *malin*, cunning? And then the evidence came to me; what needs to be exorcised, prevented, is the thread that would unfold, does unfold, when talking doesn't come along and prevent it; one has to constantly be cleaning up in order to dissuade the specific spider—the spider of being outside the consciousness of being, the verb 'to be' a non-subjectified infinitive in French, then, and outside of consciousness.

Because it's there that *le Malin*, the devil, lies, the beast forever vilified, suspected—the beast that is undoubtedly dreadful because the good lord is the Word.

So each word is learnt, repeated, in order that it is apprehended, incorporated; each word is the Host, the Host and the Maybug in the web the spider weaves, obstinately, and a spider fossil, though fossils have a hard life. And it's never too soon for the unending initiation ceremony.

In archaic societies, everything changed for children from one day to the next. They were there without truly being before the eyes of the others; they were there without being there—hope rather than reality; they were there and they were not there, between one another, this between creating both the one and the other. But these small societies had time. One day, when the moment was right and the children were a certain age, there would be an initiation that was very often savage, so to speak: a gruelling ordeal, but you do what you have to do; an ordeal that, incidentally, the children anticipated, it being the great event, and in truth a strange party, during which they would be beaten, sent away, locked up, confined, and finally, at the end of their quarantine, they would appear, in a procession. It was then, and only then, that the children were truly born.[13]

For our children, the ceremony begins immediately—an unending initiation. Do children willingly apprehend language? What an idea, as though that's all it takes, from that to words pronounced, words not particularly easy to mince, plus a garbled gobbledygook of love, and the slightest object becomes a subject—there's none other than the other, whether they be a rag, teddy bear, spoon, or anything else that comes to mind. Thus are formed good subjects: they're robust, as far as cultivated subjects go, autonomous, so to speak, citizens, ready to vote, and say whatever they like.

In French, *apprehender*, to apprehend, has veered off to become *apprendre*, to learn, by *comprendre*, comprehending. Society is in need of fully fledged, premature subject-citizens. It's got to take advantage of the anomaly that still causes us to be born as larvae in order to leave the indelible imprint, the seal of the word that makes subjects of us all, forever and practically to the core. And there is no time to lose, school awaits. And what I was made to recite when I was barely four years old was a monologue, a drunk's discourse at the statue of Napoléon; this was in honour of my godfather, who was considered an important figure; I had been named after him, and there was a family gathering down in Bergerac, thirty metres from the Dordogne; we had just learnt that my father, who I had barely glimpsed, had been killed in the war during an attack on the Biette farm near Saint-Quentin. In honour of this, my godfather came to see us, and he was to be greeted, so I had been taught a monologue: – 'Hiya . . . Poléon . . . What're you doing up there . . . ?' This while staggering about on my legs, the good premature drunk that I had to be, and it was very much a success, I understood that it was a success. . . .Monkey business?

Hanging from the pediment of a funfair stall, on the old parade ground between the Vauban citadel and the Deûle, the Pont Napoléon spanning the Deûle—there are coincidences that can't be invented—little monkeys in a parrot's cage; this was several years later, and only twenty years after that, I was there again to pick up my war uniform. It's never too soon to learn history, the same goes for the person you inherit your first name from. I'm little Fernand, *le petit*, and the large fellow, *le gros bonhomme*, is *le grand*; in honour of the large fellow, Fernand-le-Grand, Fernand-le-Petit has to recite, without mistake, his monologue for Napoléon, and he's a drunk; it's a laugh . . . Napoléon, what's that? Go on, you'll eventually learn what Napoléon is, go on; saying is never premature; the sooner you say things, the more intelligent you'll be; you say things, you repeat them: Na-po-lé-on; there you go, well done, and you make like a drunk, you make like . . . You say Napoléon and you make like a drunk; that's life. And war? Ah, right . . . the war . . . It's 1917; your father has just been killed in it.

Initiation . . . Four years old, a bit soon perhaps? Consider that little Fernand was just a year old when he heard the cannon, and not any cannon, the big one, the big, powerful cannon. . . .He was taught that it went: – 'Boom . . . ' It didn't frighten him. . . .He said: – 'Boom . . . '
He said: – 'Boom . . . ' At one year old? – 'That's right . . . He's advanced for his age. . . .'

This was up in the Nord, and now that we're in the Midi, he says Napoléon. He says:
– 'Hiya . . . Poléon . . . What're you doing up there . . . ?'

Little Fernand and then the monkeys in a parrot's cage and then the clown who happened to be a philosophy teacher—one doesn't preclude the other—and a freemason. Yet another initiation . . . and, having said that, little Fernand was a scout, a boy scout, who was nicknamed, given a totem,[14] but then that was nothing but a vague *make like*; even the war—which he was in without being in—didn't initiate him: no mark, no imprint, his skin without scars or tattoos, immunised by what he said to himself, protected by what he said to himself, protected or condemned, who knows . . .
He said to himself:
– 'What stupidity . . . '
He said to himself that this was the limit. He was mistaken. Was what he said to himself nonsense? As for the limit, he has had further news—he still gets news of the limit. And this surprises him; he has not recovered and how could he recover from a

war he was never in? He doesn't even see, on the screen, the elderly monkey locked in the parrot's cage that no doubt protects him; old habits die hard. . . .He has found something to do—his canvases. . . .Canvases that are a regular detour in the image takers' paths.

What to say? What to say to them?

– 'People are paradoxical. A brain; two hemispheres, one of which has colonised the other, and colonise is putting it mildly: one hemisphere has appropriated the other. There was a symbiosis and when one of the organisms in a symbiosis appropriates the other by profusion and phagocytosis—or any other means that comes to mind, it matters little which—what does that make? It makes the Man that we are, equipped, so to speak, with the human person, an idol like any other. And what else? Well, nothing else, or nearly nothing . . . '

The image taker has understood; he nearly has. He'll think this is where we are. He knows the human person, he even has a few in his head, so to speak; a veritable procession of them; the banners that preceded the Chicanos' protest when it went 'in the right direction'. I must have forgotten to tell him this, so I say:

– 'As César Chavez tells it, if he came to think there was a crowd in one direction and only a small group marching in the other, it was because at the head of the large procession there was a banner of the Blessed Virgin. In the other direction, no Blessed Virgin: the union's logo, which was a five-pointed star.
And if, at the age of twenty or so, I had placed this very five-pointed star in my buttonhole, it was in large part to shock my godfather, though after Poléon and the little speech, one didn't want to push things. As for his wife, she did believe—in the Blessed Virgin; there were effigies of her all over their home, at the end of the hall, in the corner of the wall; she lit up when one opened the door, and smiled, welcoming one; La Gioconda, Saint Gioconda.'

The image taker is no better off.

This is no canvas; it's me rambling on. How do you expect to frame the Chicanos' protest, the union might have disappeared or been refounded, restructured in the American manner, the Blessed Virgin having thus become a fossil—the Blessed Virgin, and the five-pointed star—and so the union is now headed by a few big shots, they're democrats and bureaucrats; how to frame the march, and at the same time, the young man, a student by trade with a red star on his lapel, who ends up at Saint Gioconda on the pretext of his being a bit lacking in character and he and the large fellow with the moustache sharing a first name . . . ?

– 'That's not all, and I say so to the image taker; large Fernand, the godfather, has a watch chain that graces his cardigan and it's the same chain, the same chain, or nearly so, as the one the philosopher used to get from his pocket and swing, in order to get what? Who knows . . . But, having said this, I'm not speaking about canvas, supposing that canvas is a tongue. I make the hole, the vacancy. I don't speak hemp; hemp is not a tongue. Images are not an apparition.'

I'm quite pleased that the word has come to me. Because does one ever know if a word will? The image taker must exorcise apparitions at all costs if ever he thinks himself to be inspired by who knows what, and thus has apparitions and projects them on a screen—apparitions or whims, it matters little; images have nothing to do with them.

Obsession? Nowadays, it's said that for art, and especially the pictorial, to be made, the painter needs to have an obsession, and why not a ghost while we're at it. To say that the spirit of the times is in need of words would be wrong; the words that are in fashion make the spirit of the times, just like the wings of a windmill make wind.

I'm talking about anchoring, and one has never seen the captain of a boat, whether or not they be a pirate, project an anchor at the end of a chain as though it were a lasso they were handling. What could be more simple than what I'm saying? One brain: two hemispheres and between the two, connections; these connections are constantly occupied. So it is that above the groove, the trench, images appear where the spider weaves, and while we're in a certain mode that could have been called human if the word were not already taken, occupied, by the fact that god is human and hence the person is; and while being—in the infinitive in French—remains entrenched, it's able to send news via these images, or via the spider's thread. Is there thus a message . . .? There is a fossil and 'fossil' doesn't mean anything, which is not a matter of ill will; animals don't mean to say anything either; the same goes for the autistic being.

And here we are, here we are again, here: I'm a regular detour in the paths of the autistic being's close presences; I have canvassed and rambled and harped on for more than fifteen years in the very shop that's a regular detour in the paths of the image takers who visit. To the extent that if they continue to visit, a rut will mark the trace of their steps.

Fifteen years ago, I said:

– 'The sign? Don't count on it. Being autistic is refractory to the idol; it's not that the autistic being is opposed to the idol, but that they don't see it; they have never seen it or understood it or anything, while every-one-of-us inevitably lugs the idol around.'

This is what I say to the image takers:

– 'Anything able to make a sign, you do without; you try to cut off the supply, that is, if there is one wherever you happen to be—signs, symbols, whims, apparitions, the whole kit and caboodle; and you don't do so by obstinate belief, which would be unbelief, because what does this matter anyway? On the banners at the head of the Chicanos' protest, the Blessed Virgin and the union logo get along well. The sign having dried up, what appear are images that don't make anything at all, least of all a sign, images of being, and there you go—images from which every-one, whoever they may be, are weaned from their earliest childhood. As for signs, every-one has seen so many made that there's a profusion of them.
What is it that folks have? They're profuse, subjugated, domesticated; they believe themselves to be the people they are—they have been mythologised, duped; they have a spider in the roof and with good reason;[15] where else do you want the spider to go? The spider ought to be spinning, weaving, between the two hemispheres. But there's no way; the spider has got to talk, talk and that's that, and say to itself, and under-say to itself, express what people say, and that says it all, and as J. P. Sartre said—and he was absolutely in favour—when he first saw the S' slung over the shoulder, fortunately we had *Les Temps modernes* between us, and not the film by Charlie Chaplin, but the journal, the journal to be made, and what could be more Vatican-like, as in the church, than the chapels of artists?'

Canvassing is a tough métier, as it's true that I harp on, just like a priest, the priest fossil that I am, every priest being the fossil form of the priest of old who was not a priest, but a chief, or I don't know, a shaman, and before that, the elderly person, or the halfwit who soliloquised; every society is in need of an individual who provides this service; the priest is much more of a fossil than he appears, with his gestures and ritual words; the ritual doesn't mean anything; he sings, but is this singing his voice being modulated and finding its way? The right hemisphere; because this is very much at the limit, the limit of the symbolic, of the gestures and humming that are those of the autistic being. If I write this, nobody will give a damn, and if the camera captures a priest while he's officiating, what will be seen, on the screen, is a rather old-fashioned priest, and there you have it. Who will see the fossil and the autistic being? No one.

The Man that we are is paradoxical, but this is not seen.[16]

Notes

1 'Les fossiles ont la vie dure. À propos d'image' was written in August of 1982 and first published in 2021 as part of *Camérer. À propos d'images*, Paris, L'Arachnéen, 2021.

2 La place de la République in Armentières, though Deligny likely confused the date, as he resided in Paris in 1937 and moved to the town in 1939.

3 Deligny's mate uses the idiomatic expression, '*on lui a fait la peau*', which mentions *la peau*, 'the skin', connecting, for the French reader, his words to the scrap of the priest's skin he keeps in his wallet.

4 Here again, Deligny makes use of a variant of the idiomatic expression, '*Il y a laissé sa peau*', literally, 'He left his skin behind'.

5 André Malraux and Boris Peskine, directors, *Espoir: Sierra de Teruel (Days of Hope)*, Les Productions André Malraux and Productions Corniglion-Molinier, 1945.

6 The term 'chicanos' has for some time been used by Mexican Americans, irrespective of how they entered the United States and their country of birth.

7 Deligny writes, '*c'est d'images que je "cause", ou plutôt de ce qui pourrait, éventuellement, les causer, étant bien entendu qu'elles ne causent pas*'. In so doing, he makes use of the two main meanings of the verb *causer*: 'to chat' in the first instance, and thereafter (and earlier in the paragraph), 'to cause'.

8 *Un métier* has two meanings in French: 'a loom' and that of the loanword commonly used in English. Deligny plays with the ambiguity in meanings here and then goes on to differentiate between the two in the following paragraphs.

9 Deligny's neologism, *l'à-faire*, rendered here literally as 'to-do', and *l'affaire*, are homophones, such that the French reader would understand that the adorned is a 'matter' for the image taker.

10 Deligny uses the idiomatic expression '*j'en mettrais ma main au feu*', literally, 'I would put my hand in fire', which is roughly equivalent in meaning to 'I would bet my life on it'. The latter loses the hand in question, however, which in the French reappears in '*témoin de première main*', 'first-hand witness'.

11 Though the verb *investiguer* does appear to exist, its use is less common than that of the nouns for the act and the person.

12 Deligny describes Moustapha Al Akkad's film *The Lion of the Desert* (Anchor Bay Entertainment, 1981), the details of which he learnt on the France Inter radio programme at 1:00 p.m. on August 3, 1982.

13 In the original manuscript, this paragraph is followed by an incomplete sentence that was omitted from the translation for the sake of coherency. The fragment reads '*de tous ces rites qui sont bons pour des primitifs demeurés*': 'of all those rites that are good for primitive half-wits'.

14 In France, boy scouts are given a 'totem', the name of an animal that their troop feels represents them.

15 *Avoir une araignée dans le plafond*, translated here literally as 'they have a spider in the roof', is an idiomatic expression used similarly to the English idiom 'they have bats in the belfry', the 'roof' or 'belfry' in question being the head.

16 The manuscript ends on the following unfinished line, which reads: '*Karl Marx, de cette espèce qui se dit humaine, il ne savait pas trop quoi foutre. Alors*'—'Karl Marx, of the species that considers itself humane, didn't really know what the hell to do. So'.

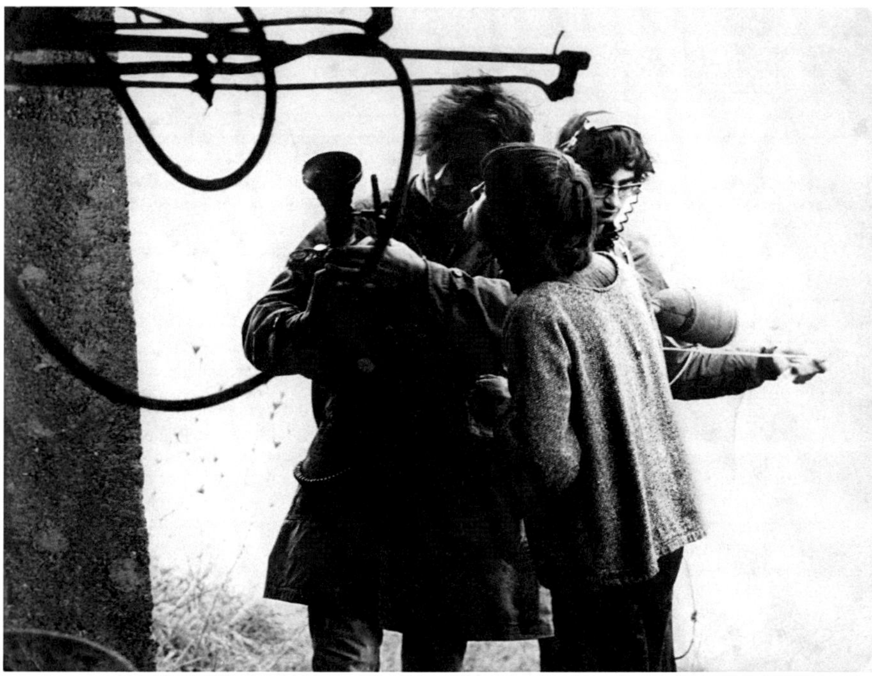

Shooting of *That Kid, There*, around 1974. Renaud Victor on the camera with Janmari and Guy Canonge in the background.

Camering [1978-1983][1]

Filmer, to film, seems to me an odd verb. When it's a matter of writing a book, *un livre*, one doesn't say booking, or *livrer*. And the verb *peindre*, to paint, is used and not *tableauter*, from *un tableau*, a painting. Here one sees that when it comes to cinema, the final product prevails and becomes a verb. One says *raboter*, to plane a wooden plank, and not *planchelisser*, *une planche* being the noun for that plank.

Since it's a matter of using an instrument called a camera, why doesn't one say camering? It's true that working with a microscope is not called microscoping. But the microscope doesn't produce anything other than a certain way of seeing, while the camera is an image mill; however, contrary to the windmill, the images don't make it go round, or *tourner*. The camera rolls on its own, and what's said is: '*On tourne*'—'We're rolling'.

On? One, in English. Indefinite personal pronoun, third person, fixed, in French always functions as the subject. Could one not have put this any better? It would appear that *on* is pronounced 'om', which comes from *homo*. '*Silence, l'homme tourne*'—'Quiet, man's rolling'. That has an altogether different feel to it.

In the word camera, the chamber is visible. The word that follows in the dictionary is *camérier*, or chamberlain: 'an officer in the pope's chambers.' Most cineastes would be very surprised to be called a chamberlain, or worse, a *camériste*, or chambermaid: 'a woman who attended to a princess.' Might that princess be the reigning ideology?

If I hang these remarks on the nail of a surprising infinitive, it's perhaps to indicate that the camera can make something quite different from a film, just as writing can be done without the direct object that is called a book. But then what's the point of activating that mechanism responsible for subterfuge, subterfuge made possible by a fault in our seeing apparatus: retinal persistence? Our gaze slides over the jerks and we're gone with the movement reproduced. And then the sound joins in, and the colour, which gets to be a bit much.

We're there, you might say, as if we were there, so what's the use of this equipment? You need only look calmly out a window, or not, if the urge comes over you to go see the summit of the Himalayas. Hence the disappearance of a seventh art as overloaded with means as someone who's filthy rich and commits suicide because of the ennui that comes with having so much.

What happened to us—and I can say that it took place the other way around, or nearly so—was that we were lacking in means to such an extent that all we had was a 16 mm camera and nothing more. The camera didn't collect sound, or images, truth be told, for want of film—something to think about, if only in an idle moment.

Ten years later, we had ten hours of images rolled up in tin cans, and we needed only see them to know what was inside. We didn't know what was on the reels because we didn't have an apparatus with which to project the images. And, once again, the funds lacking, montage and audio mixing were pushed far back. It would take us another ten years.

Prior to that, I got to know other aspects of cinema, if only because I was a delegate at Travail et Culture, where this entailed the green canvas duffel bags into which the film club's programme was piled. And what sometimes happened was that the bag was not there, at the train station. Sometimes the film *was* there and it was the audience who was not at the screening.

And so, still ten years prior, since I was the one who wrote the film reviews in the student paper, I received rectangles of Bristol board inviting me to screenings that took place in the morning in cinemas that were almost empty, so much so that I could watch the film at a distance, from the back of the room, or up high, on the balcony, or up close, right in front of the screen.

I also happened to circulate movies shot in a North Vietnam that was grappling with the Americans. Sometimes, there were ten or so country folk in the back room of the pub and I was transported to the time of the magic lantern. One could believe, with a bit of effort, that it was the first time they had seen a film. And as for me, I saw the same film ten or twenty times.

If one says that memories shift along a string, like prayer beads—and not all of them are, far from it—then they remain alive forever. I let go of memories from films I grappled with as they were being made, disinclined as I am to watch a film I'm involved with. I avoid the ordeal that is waiting for images I don't see coming. Where have they gone? And I wait. And they don't come because they're not there. But if they're not there, how can it be that I wait for them? Could it be that they're camered in my head, and there alone? Either that or the images were too beautiful, so striking that the film could not handle them. Perhaps it's that they disappeared during montage because they interfered with the course of history,[2] that they led nowhere, or that one would wonder where they had come from, what they were doing there.

History. We're perhaps at the point where filming and camering diverge. I remain amenable to the chance occurrence that placed in my hands the book in which were found the three lines I don't dare write myself. I began writing this text yesterday morning. Yesterday afternoon, I half-opened a book by Jacques Berque: *Arabies* (*Arabias*).[3]
'Take away the sense of history (a sense to be criticised, renewed, it's true) and what reason would there be to combat racism, exploitation, or simply incoherence?'
History?
'Knowledge of, or relationship between, past events and facts relative to the evolution of humanity that are worthy or considered worthy of memory.'
'Accounts of actions, of events real or imagined.'

There remains natural history which, when I was young, was called object lessons, the objects having no history. Indeed. If I were a cineaste, I would dream of camering the path of an iceberg and its thaw and the succession of changes in its appearance, at first a mountain that separates from an ice field, and the effort involved in its breaking off, and the sounds; this being altogether different from whatever actors might jabber on about; and the mist, and the seabirds, and how long it lasts, that mass of which only an ice floe the size of a fist will remain, and then nothing; nothing other than the sea. The event camered in real time, weeks would be needed to render it, to reproduce it; permanent cinema. Nothing but the iceberg on the screen for weeks. Those who wished to go see it would do so, even if only every now and then, to see where things stand, to see what remains, of the iceberg. The sense of history that we have because it was given to us would be refreshed.

It may be that upon renewing this 'sense', which we clearly see is not the sixth art, or the seventh, since it owes everything to what could be called ethnic memory, the camera becomes the instrument that arrives at the right time, and let's hope it's not the last time it does, if we imagine where history will take us if we let it, fretting as would a cub atop the iceberg I mentioned above. We fret, that's for certain. But what is history? It's that which can be narrated. It's the screenplay.

It may well be that as soon as it's a matter of the making of a film—that necessary prerequisite—an obligation arises, it being the railroad switch that determines whether one goes about filming or camering.

How many cineastes are no more than something of a failed writer, given that their vague intentions have no objective, what with the objective not being the subject, but the instrument, the sentence itself. They would know what to say if they knew how. In the absence of that *how*, which doesn't come to them, it's the camera they make use of, an orthopaedic instrument that comes to the rescue of their linguistic ineptitude. It's there that the distinctiveness of what they would camer disappears.

From that time in my existence when, once or twice a week, I went to see films in cinemas that were empty, or nearly so, what remains is something like a crux of confusion. Among the films shown, there were the good ones, and the bad ones. I spoke of the good films, so that one went to see them and perhaps also for the pleasure of reworking, in my manner, the reviews I had read.

In those days, people went to the cinema like the Greeks did the theatre in times past. It was a question of tradition and a weekly ritual; the interest in what happened on the screen was entirely secondary.[4] But that was not the crux of my perplexity. As to the films I spoke of, I might remember the title and the director and the actors. But when it comes to the other films, the bad ones, the ones I no longer remember, it's clear that the images remain. But who knows where? They're surely scattered all over, like shards of metal in the flesh of a soldier of times past.

Here one sees that there could be two types of memory, which is what I believe: one where language is sovereign, and another that in a way resists symbolic domestication, that is somewhat aberrant, and that allows itself to be struck by that which doesn't mean anything, if one understands being struck to be a shock that leaves an imprint.

Camering would entail respecting that which doesn't mean anything, doesn't say anything, doesn't address anyone; in other words, that which eludes the symbolic domestication without which there would be no history—whether individual or collective—for a lack of consciousness.

In addition to an ethnic memory that bears the deep imprint of exploitation and racism and the incoherencies that seek, obstinately, to reproduce, there would thus be another memory that nourishes itself on what it gleans from here and there. To say that this memory is poor would be an understatement. It's literally forgotten, which, as far as a memory goes, is ironic. Perhaps it should be called differently. In times past, it was a custom in the homes of the rich, that is to say, in the homes of those who were the most domesticated, to have a bowl ready for the vagabond, just in case.

It happens that in the richest of films, the most sumptuous, there are leftovers. The directors of these films are impregnated with the sense they want to give their history for the edification of mass audiences, and so it is that there's something to nourish the poor woman, who's deaf and mute, and who doesn't understand the reason behind the historical-sentimental orgy. To say that she doesn't fall for it would be an understatement. She doesn't even see the bait. What I mean is that deprived of the sense of history, while everybody cries, she has herself a good laugh; while everybody laughs, she cries—but it's not heard. It's discreet, the human there hides, forbidden since time began, since history began.

Here it becomes clear that camering would be something other than filming.

Yesterday, I saw, on the small TV that belongs to us, to those of us who live close to autistic children—it so happens that we have the use of a video camera—I saw D., who's soon to be nine, absorbed in taking a good look at the hand that, for us, is his, and moving it around in the water. If I say taking a good look, it's to avoid saying that he watched the hand, if watching is understood to be our way of seeing, the way of those of us who have a sense of history, even if it's only our own.

Strange TV that we can rewatch, every now and then, to see what's going on with us; we can rewatch the TV and we can watch it, because that we consists of those of us who live kilometres away from each other, and who thus don't see each other live, except via the intervention that is the small TV that's become common memory, and that enables us to ask ourselves what we're offering for others to see, those who don't care the least bit about what our histories are doing.

The bowl is set down, even if we don't know how and with what to fill it. We would have to film that about us which eludes us, that which is not seen (by the self); that *self* being what's taken as the subject of history, of history strictly speaking, and of one's own history in particular.

To such an extent that I could have called this text 'In search of lost images', which would have made for quite a nice title.

It would have been about the images that are cut during montage, like wood shavings, or worse, those that are not recorded to begin with.

One need only imagine, during the shooting of a normal film, produced in a normal fashion and put together according to the norms, all the images, the most beautiful images, and by far the most moving ones, that, we discover—for reasons unbeknown to us—are deliberately not included.

Camering would be recording these images, because one never knows, because one will see.

I happened to hear talk of *découpage*. The dictionary says that what's involved is poultry, cake, or meat, and suggests we look up chopping, carving, quartering. And so the time has come for us to talk about theatre and cinema. I clearly see a producer who requires a director to first proceed to quarter his project. Later, if the pieces are good and fit together well, all that remains is racing the horse and hoping it brings back the Palme d'Or. And why not? It happens.

It's remarkable that those children who have shown themselves to be resistant to symbolic domestication watch us living, us. More often than not they remain seated. In their posture and their appearance one finds those of a person at the cinema or watching television. They watch us as though we were the protagonists of a television series that has no ending, and more often than not, it's the water they go see. And there, their gaze comes alive, and their body. Becoming water seems to them more tempting than becoming like us. Some of them are amazed, and that is understandable.

So what about camering?

Camering would entail making the most of that small grinding chamber in order to do a bit of squinting at something other than the very course of occurrences that are what they are, experienced by people, experienced being an overstatement, which is what one says about a fictional film.

Anything else?
As to the things that move us, that stir us, we have no idea why they do. They evade history, with or without a capital H, but without them history would not be what it is.

Squinting is really a nice verb. There would be two *oculare*, two oculars, and not at all to see in relief; two oculars like there are two types of memory, to such an extent that the *on qui tourne*—the one who shoots—would have something like one eye that lingers in search of what's purely human, even if it's only scraps, in addition to and beyond the scene screenplayed.

One needs to invent a camera that squints.

Notes

1 The final of the three 'Camérer' pieces included in this collection was written between 1978 and 1983. It first appeared in the 4th issue of *Caméra/Stylo* in September of 1983. It was called 'Camérer #1' in *Camérer. À propos d'images*, Paris, L'Arachnéen, 2021.

2 Deligny writes '*le déroulement de l'histoire*', which could be read as 'the course of history' or 'the story's development'.

3 Mirèse Akar and Jacques Berque, *Arabies: entretiens avec Mirèse Akar*, Paris, Stock, 1978.

4 The French reads, *'l'intérêt de ce qui (se) passait sur l'écran étant tout à fait secondaire'*. By placing the reflexive pronoun *se* in brackets, Deligny works two possible meanings into the sentence: *se passer*, 'to happen'—as it has been translated here—and *passer*, which could be understood as 'to pass through'.

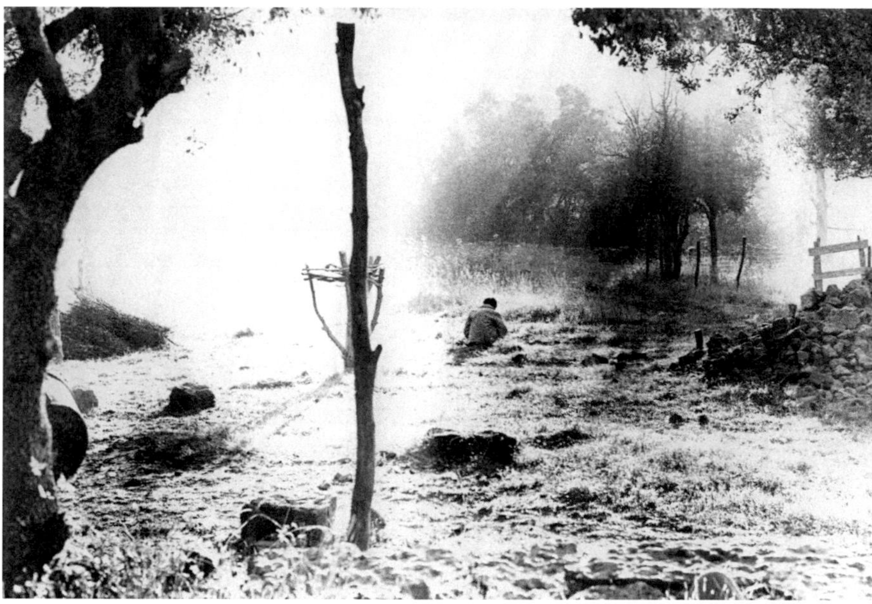

Le Serret living area, end of 1970s.

The Distinctiveness of the IMAGEs [1988][1]

The image is distinct in being an image.
In the place of language, there is only language, in whatever form it may take.
The image does not become language.
Language is not transformed into image.

There may be symbiosis between language and image.
But symbiosis is association, not confusion, and one that is lasting and mutually beneficial.
The Man that we are is lichen, alga and fungus, that is, in this case, image and language.
That said, what becomes of the image, if we admit that the image eludes being language?

It's a question of language approaching what it might be like to be an image, of language believing that it grasps the image, understands it, assimilates it.
This having been done—and it's a decoy—there remains the image, still just as enduring; the fungus didn't appropriate the alga; the Man—that we are—is lichen.

*
* *

If I write that Man is lichen, lichen in this case is not image.
It's a plant or, to put it better, an organism made from an alga and a fungus; perhaps a promising monster, as they say in biology.
Likewise human beings, who are promising—if they happen to persist instead of destroying themselves?

*
* *

It can also happen that language flows into the image; it's thus that the being—human that we are—becomes a tree.
Believing is enough.

*
* *

I have sometimes said:

– 'Image is what is not seen (by the self).'

This comment didn't make the task any easier for the image taker who happened to be here.

That said, I suggested he regard his camera as not being able to take movement, movement being what is seen.

I had gone to tell him that image and movement were of the same nature, movement—in cinema—being caused by what is called retinal persistence.

Who knows what 'persistence' the image—that everyone sees even though it is not there—develops from.

*

* *

What I say to the image taker:

– 'If the image is not there in—in or on—the film, there is no point looking to take—so to speak—images, since it's understood that images will capture themselves, as it were, just like flies on pre-war sticky paper.'

You just need to find the glue.

But the image taker doesn't want these images to be dead; the images must be very much alive, all enduring.

And that's quite understandable.

I calmly explain to him that what I said about the flypaper—apropos of images—is merely a terribly unrefined analogy and nothing to be offended at; between a film—especially the film he foresees—and flypaper, there is only the tape form in common—between that paper and the film; and perhaps also the fact that, just like with images, flies circle around looking for you, but to capture them you have to swat them with a folded-up newspaper.

*

* *

On this film undertaken in common—there are four or five of us—I'm the artisan, like the three or four others, and everyone does their bit.

My part—my bit—is to hammer out a few words:

– 'The image is distinct in being an image.'

I'm a prayer wheel, and with the utmost respect, nowhere does it say that images will allow themselves to be captured.

*

* *

This is what I say to the image taker:

– 'When you talk about the image, what are you talking about?'

He falls silent; and yet he has read plenty of works and texts and articles that talk about this alone.

At first, he had a vague idea of what the image could be, but now even that idea has vanished.

He's on the right path; the way is clear.

*

* *

As far as I'm concerned, the image doesn't give a damn about language, and the role of language is to exterminate the image.

Now we're in a fine mess.

It remains to think of the precedent, of the forgotten arch-ancestor, the lichen.

The alga doesn't give a damn about the fungus, and the fungus would certainly eat up the alga.

The fact is that they live in symbiosis, and this is lichen.

The cineastes that we are should celebrate lichen like others do Christmas.

*

* *

I knew one—individual of this species of ours—who would sit in front of a screen while a film was being projected and see nothing—it seemed—perhaps not even movement.

Who knows. . . .That 'he' had no use of language, none at all, which is to say much less than the slightest deaf-mute.

Or else he would see images, images no matter where he looked; so what good is a screen?

*

* *

This cineaste—among others—has seen so many films that when he makes one—a film—whoever sees it says to themself that they have already seen it. . . .

So? The image may need to be reiterated.

*

* *

If I make a film in 1963, I frame—so to speak—in the style of Soviet cineastes in 1927; and the film is—possibly—a masterpiece.

*
* *

Some put love at the heart of anything they do—as a manner of speaking.
Everyone has their own manner of doing things; mine is to talk of spite. I have to do it to do anything.
To talk image is, for me, to fight—desperately—against the language ONE uses without discernment.

*
* *

I fear—quite seriously—that as a result of hearing that they must communicate, talk, etc . . . etc . . . children will become mute.

*
* *

If our friend WITT. says something that is barely founded when he describes ethics as the desire that drives us—we, the Man-that-we-are—to run against the boundaries of language, then the image I'm talking about is ethical.[2]
The image would then be at the very core of ethics.

*
* *

We need only consider an anthill . . .
We still have to get to it; what can be seen are ants and a few holes scattered here and there.
If we believe those who have seen it from up close, every species of ant has its own anthill that's distinct from the anthill of neighbouring species.
An image of this anthill would thus need to be made, but then where would this image be—in the meantime? The same goes for spiders or beavers or termites.
And as far as we're concerned, where can the image be found? On the screen, no doubt?

*
* *

It may be that making a film is a quest for what the IMAGE could be, this quest being the work common to all those who make film.

*
* *

Could it be that the slightest image is common—to everyone in our species?
As far as I'm concerned, that could certainly be the case.

*
* *

Image is that without which language could not be.
That said, image doesn't become language and language doesn't become image.

*
* *

ONE talks about a style full of imagery, when talking about a writer.
Why not; ONE says plenty of other things.

*
* *

If I see myself—on a screen—is it an image?
If so, is this 'myself'—from 'I see myself'—thus an image?
Here I am, overwhelmed at what I am and at being an image.
The same thing happens in radiography—I want to talk about X-rays—where ONE can see 'me'—but what a strange 'me' that is. You would have to be very clever to recognise yourself. But where is that 'me' from the screen? On the screen? He's only projected there, from a film. Is he therefore on this film—this 'he' being 'me', let us remember? Not really; in capturing me, the other day, the camera didn't capture any of me, that I know of. And here, are we grappling with the mystery of the anthill whose image is in the head of the little hymenoptera? But does the insect have, strictly speaking, a head? In the joints of the little nodes of its nervous system, or in the earth perhaps; or in the heavens . . .

*
* *

This is why the image taker is often perplexed. . . .
Everything I say only increases this perplexity.
I regret it, but I would regret it even more if I let him believe all the sententious nonsense, of very dubious worth, that he may have read or heard.

*
* *

This nonsense—apropos of images—is very profuse, disparate, and contradictory.
I have on occasion heard images, *images*, talked about—on the radio perhaps—and believed that 'what' was being talked about was cheese, *fromage*, the misunderstanding lasting a fair while.
If I were a carnival barker, I would speak—as well as any other—of creamy images, and even of the dough, of that dough that images are made from. It's a marvel that cinema has not disappeared, suffocated under this pile of words.
It has not disappeared at all. People even say that the more we talk about it, the better it gets, regardless of what we say.
This would prove that language won't have—won't ever have—image.
Lichen persists—despite everything.

*
* *

Once upon a time there was a jackdaw, a western jackdaw.
It was impossible to film what was in its head.
And what a shame, because there, it seems, was pure image.

*
* *

Just the other day, the image taker tried to get me to say whether the fossil that keeps me company—it's undoubtedly of a fish—could be called: image. And this under the pretext that the fossil is, in his eyes, a masterpiece.
After that, he asked me whether this fish bone, which was traced on rock over thousands and thousands of years, was art or not.
I was rather stunned.
What did I say? That I was not in possession of the truth that he asked of me, that we would have to debate with each other; I was at a loss for words, and even at a loss for all good sense.

He preferred to go back to film; the everyperson can't do it all.

*

* *

You know *le réalisateur,* the director, of a film coming out. He's a pretentious nitwit who only thinks about money.
And throughout the film that you—nonetheless—go and see, by chance, are images, and images to your heart's content, like swallows on a telephone wire the evening before they migrate.
That's life.
You shouldn't try to do as much—as this *réalisateur*; and as life.

*

* *

You've got to do something else.
And in doing something else, what you do is the same thing—because the others, too, those who came before you, wanted to do something else.
That said, in doing something else, they wanted their oeuvre to be recognised.
But how can you recognise something else when you have never seen it?

*

* *

Before—I mean before my time—people went to the cinema for the sake of it; the film—whatever it was—being merely a pretext.
Now, you go to see such-and-such a film, and you end up in the cinema.

*

* *

I would say, about the image, what Henri Michaux said about the night:
 – 'It stirs . . . '
and it's a whole world.
I should write:
 – 'The image stir [*sic*] . . . '

(the words)

*

* *

The image only exists as a myriad.

*
* *

The part chance plays in the image is as decisive as the part language plays in the intention.
Here one sees that making a film—so to speak, since it's not a question of acting if acting is understood as reacting—takes 'a circuitous and tortuous route carved by adaptations evolved for different reasons, and fortunately suited to later needs.'
I take these lines from the biologist S. J. Gould who thus described the 'fortuitous series of accidents' on which our existence as living beings depends.[3]
It's thanks to a succession of cataclysms that we are—here.

*
* *

The image is due to chance and has a very long history, a never-ending history; a chain of disasters has as a whole cleared the path so that the unexpected image may emerge.

*
* *

The image is not taken.
It happens; we still have to erase what we once believed indispensable, erase again, erase ceaselessly.
Then the image will be glimpsed.
That is what Giacometti did—and he was not a cineaste.
The other day, I was telling the image taker that it had occurred to me to make a movie without film.
We had a camera and so it was understood that a movie would be made.
And the movie began to be made—while we waited for the film—every one of us there becoming another, the other who they would be if the movie were made.
The image then had a tremendous time and proliferated due to the fact that there was nothing to trap it.
No film, no sticky paper.

*
* *

All oeuvres—including those of cinema—depend on innumerable coincidences. If the image(s) taker waits for the coincidences he could be waiting for a long time.

*

* *

Language is learnt.
The image is always already there.

*

* *

I once knew an image taker who went crazy.
He was convinced that he had the image(s) in his head and was surprised that when he looked at the screen there was nothing there.

*

* *

In his last work, a professor at the Collège de France, a renowned scholar, wrote that as far as the Man-that-we-are is concerned, the memory of education substitutes for the memory of the species.[4]
To substitute means to take the place in order to assume the same role.
That the memory of the species and the memory of education play the same role is a surprising notion.
And the declaration that the memory of education can be identified with the memory of the species is even more surprising.
If the memory of the species and the image are in some way of the same stock, it's easier to understand why the image—distinctly speaking—has disappeared—this said in the eyes of language.

*

* *

When asked why he makes music, a renowned composer, a famous conductor, could reply that he doesn't know at all.
But he replies:
– 'I make music to say . . . '
If it's to say something, speaking suffices.

*

* *

I wonder where this inflation of language is heading.
– 'Here we are, ONE says, in the era of the image . . . '
And what is the image for?
– 'To express oneself . . . '
Who knows what this self, this S'—that would appear in the image—might be.

*
* *

That the image is not seen (by the SELF) doesn't mean that it's invisible, but that the SELF doesn't see anything there—as long as the image is there.

*
* *

Remove the self from language, and it becomes disjointed.
Likewise, if we believe our friend WITT., if you extirpate the intention, it collapses.

*
* *

The image is there, it's always already there.
There may be times when it is not seen, when it's not seen by this SELF.
But by another?
And if it's never seen, is this not proof that it doesn't exist?

*
* *

So for the image taker(s), it would be a question of IMAGE being seen.
If IMAGE is within the purview of the memory of the species, it must be very common.
What makes every-one different—from the other—is perhaps—in addition to all that one learnt while the other was learning something else—that for one, language is thicker—as might be said about a layer—than for the other.

*
* *

You should have seen the care with which this scholar-researcher looked for traces of the customary of a minor people who died out thousands of years ago.
We were stunned, and stunned again when the same person professed that the memory of education substitutes for the memory of the species.

*
* *

To the detriment of which all progress is established . . .
This is not vague nostalgia.
It's in this detriment that—those who search—find the signs of the progress to come.

*
* *

In the absence of the memory of education—what happens is that the memory of the species—rich in image(s)—allows the human-being to spot—and thus react—opportunely.
But spot what?
Everything but the SELF—the self spotting itself.

*
* *

Even in the cinema, there can occasionally be image(s) on the screen.
ONE is stunned.

*
* *

I learnt write at a very young age . . .
I wonder why 'to' would be placed there.

*
* *

Instead of image, better to simply write i.
This is what I say to the image taker. We would no longer be encumbered by the word-that-means.

*
* *

Nothing worse, for the user, than all these words that mean.
If words really mean, let them say so.
And we'll go fishing, or watch the images go by from the top of the church tower.

*
* *

The fact that I write—very conscientiously—the image(s) brings to mind clones, those groups of genetically similar individuals that come from a single organism . . . etc.
In this case, what becomes of the organism? Is it the individual, or is it the species?

*
* *

Whatever it may seem, I'm fiercely individualistic; the subject is what fellow beings, who are similar to each other, depend on.

*
* *

Since the appearance of language . . .
Because language had to appear at a given moment.
Given by whom? A good number of religions, immensely disparate as they are, reply:
– By God.
Those who don't have—religion—or hardly do, need to think that language was given (to us) by the greatest of chances and myriad coincidences.

*
* *

'No analysis, no explanation, subtle though it may be, can replace the sensation one feels at the SIGHT of a work of art; what is above all indispensable to me, is to SEE.'
I fully understand; but what about music?

*
* *

It's true that IMAGE(s) seems reserved for SEEING, whereas IMAGE(s) is hearing, or feeling, or whatever else comes to mind that, when perceived by any of the senses—and often many of the senses at once—could be.

*
* *

It's a question here of the image taker and the person who writes reaching an agreement on the rigours of a practice.
IMAGEs taken?
I prefer to say camering, since it entails the camera, and not filming—which is said just as one does nailing.

*
* *

It's a question of creating . . .
Creating IMAGEs?
Creating the conditions necessary—and, perhaps, sufficient—for IMAGEs to exist.
But if the IMAGEs is not seen (by the self)?
It's heard, it's smelled, it's distinguished, it's felt.
The images ONE talks about are (of) language.

*
* *

The IMAGEs doesn't let itself be said; what is IMAGEs can be spotted; ONE doesn't know what to say . . . and yet. . . .

*
* *

For a few days now, on my workbench, I have had a ray within hand's reach.
A ray?
– Painted on bark, by an Australian Aborigine.
It was the image taker who brought it to me. He told himself that I would be happy to see it. At this moment, it is—to me—the most beautiful work of art in the world; and this moment could last years.

*
* *

One should not believe; one should never believe and, that said, as far as I'm aware, I believe this.
This?
Who knows.

*
* *

It's impossible for me to say what ONE doesn't say.

*
* *

It's true that the IMAGEs can't be learnt. Hence the fact that, since language has existed, the IMAGEs has fallen into disuse.

*
* *

It seems to me that Karl Marx noted that from the moment the individual born of exchange appeared, a whole mode of thinking—one might say world, *monde*, instead of mode—was no longer useful, disappeared.
He noted in the margin: Come back to this.
Now this, I believe.
You have to come back to this—obstinately.

*
* *

Since language has existed—and all that it allows: the detriment.

*
* *

A mode of thinking, and it's a whole world. Which doesn't mean that the world is only a mode of thinking.

*
* *

ONE uses what ONE has:
- Oneself

*
* *

What does our friend WITT. say?
- 'Language doesn't allow us to get out of IT—the very least of IT being the world of language.'

Because language is a whole world.
Hence the IMAGE(s) and its necessity, in order to deal with the excesses of absolute exclusivity—because exclusivity is power.

*
* *

What work does the social worker do, social work? Certainly not. This would take at the very least a revolution. So what to do—as it's necessary to work—by which I mean, who to lay into? The subject.

*
* *

It can be said that the IMAGEs is tacit.
It remains to specify what tacit entails that is not keeping silent.

*
* *

Our friend WITT. talks about those arrangements of the tacit without which language would just be throat noise.
But he treats the IMAGEs like a slave of all word.
This is why I left the word where it was, full of hidden meanings; put otherwise, a lot of language.

*
* *

All words are (of) language.
This is why I take IMAGEs, and lay it outside.
Like one might do a king or a bishop ready to intervene in a game of draughts.

*
* *

A certain memory is of having.
Another is of being.

*
* *

The IMAGEs leads its little existence.
This is—it seems to me—undeniable.
And the commotion is incessant.

*
* *

If language is intention, it should not be necessary to say that a dog—a dog and all that lives—wants—anything. But then, how to say it?
Here we are, provided with a language that is uniquely our own.
That said, ONE makes it say everything, if not directly, then at least by allusion.
Some make it their speciality to tell others what THEY mean.
But who is the THEY in question?

*
* *

It could be that the Man-that-we-are has as many memories as a dromedary has stomachs.

*
* *

So the IMAGEs?
A certain memory is of learning.
And the others? They would be of being.

*
* *

For those who have not learnt language, 'it' is not there—and therefore has no hands; it could be human.
These hands—which ONE says are one's own—are of a human being.
Here it's seen that the sense of ownership comes from afar; from the intervention of *to have* in the language.
Is there a—human—language that doesn't have *to have* among its primordial verbs?

*
* *

Our friend WITT. tells us:
– 'Of course, the image has no intention; but it's with the image that we do . . . '
I understand.
And he adds:
– 'But if having an intention, and meaning, are things that are produced with the image, I don't see why they should be linked to a person.'
And it's true, it seems to me, that one of the flipsides of language is to be utopian, to the extent that we wonder what the person who speaks is doing in there.

*
* *

We see the importance of the image for our friend WITT.; it's at the core of intention—that without which intention would not take—so to speak—place; intention being thought—said—and thus of language.

*
* *

Our friend WITT. again:
– 'If it goes without saying that people take pleasure in their own imagination, one must recall that what they imagine is not comparable with a painted image or a plastic model; rather, it's a complicated image, made of heterogeneous elements: words and images among others.'
But what does the image taker become in this imbroglio? He's lost.
This is why I anchor myself to the distinctiveness of the IMAGEs.

*
* *

The distinctiveness of the IMAGEs—it seems to me—for if the image is understood to be what our friend WITT. says it is, namely, a word full of all that comes to ONE's mind, then we're not yet out of the woods.
Once upon a time there was a snail that had just died—something which no doubt happens to snails, just as it does to others.
The mollusc, strictly speaking, passed away. There remained the shell, which filled up with a bit of everything and just about anything.
Thus filled, the shell returned to take its place in the dictionary, bursting with meaning—if everything that ONE had put in the shell can be called meaning.
Now, if the image taker endeavours to project these images, it should not come as a surprise if cinema falls into disuse.

*

* *

It's said that a word can be empty of meaning.
Which—ONE says—nature abhors—and the nature of people in particular.

*

* *

No image, no intention, our friend WITT. tells us.
And without intention can there be IMAGEs? Image is the word that ONE says, and IMAGEs would be what makes that word distinct.
IMAGEs, it seems to me, has no intention.

*

* *

The image taker thus holds in their hands an apparatus that takes shots at such a rate that movement will appear in the eyes of the viewer.
Is it then a question of appearing or seeming to appear?
Does the viewer create the movement?
Create? That's shooting from nothingness or realising something that didn't exist before.
The apparatus—held by the image taker—shoots images and it's the viewer who shoots the movement; but from where?

*

* *

In the beginning, god created movement and, later, the camera; who knows why . . .
The same is true of the image, which had existed for a good long time when the camera was invented; and why? Why do it?
Cineastes have asked themselves this for as long as they have existed; the answers are disparate.

*
* *

Searching for the distinctiveness of the IMAGEs is a way to not get caught up in the word, the word itself.
And what our friend WITT. says about this deserves our attention:
– 'The way we feel the experience of the image, makes it reality for us.'

The image taker is lost; and I too get lost.
I suggest that we fall back on the cinematic image, which is a particular image in that it needs a whole slew of apparatuses and screens.
A particular image, then, which has nothing to do with wall paintings or speech rate.
Nothing except that it's human.
What necessity does the Man-that-we-are—and which we always have been—what necessity to project the IMAGEs?
For wall paintings are projected; pro? Forwards, the dictionary tells us, in favour of . . . and, all things considered, in support of.
But of what?
Who knows what the human being who traced a buffalo on the wall of some cave was a supporter of.
Or the Australian Aborigine who trace-painted the ray on bark that can be seen on my workbench. What were they a supporter of?

*
* *

Could it be some project, a project common to every individual of this species of ours?
Imagine the number of supporters who have lived and live this common project . . .
Some think—perhaps—that this project—which is one of IMAGEs—occurs in language, tints it, soaks in it. . . .I don't think so at all. . . .
And that is a choice, one so radical that it has cost me a good number of supporters—'me' being a certain approach.
They were attached to language.
Does this mean I'm not attached to it?

I'm alert to not being wholly attached—or understood.
And yet, I would like very much to be heard, if only by the image taker.

*
* *

This is what I say to him:

– 'It's not a matter of understanding—what I say—but of hearing it.'

If folks were happy to hear—language—without seeking so much to understand or believe, the earth could start to turn backwards, I mean in the other direction, which would be the right one.

*
* *

The image taker brings me a photo of a Brazilian kid—he's from the Maghreb, I should say, but no matter—who has just found a rope, the very rope that held hay loads and timber loads.[5]
He knows the attraction I feel for all ropes.
From the rope to the knot, there is only one step, and from the knot to the hanged man, one more step.
Over the past few days, I finished reading the translation of a book by Traven: – *The Rebellion of the Hanged*.[6]
And over twenty years ago now, I made a feature film in which the hero was a knot, the true hero; there were other characters too—including one who disappeared at the start of the film.
There were four or five of us around the camera.
A grown-up kid was there; he didn't know anything about the knot.
Since his birth—fifteen years prior—he had certainly seen knots tied; before his eyes, so to speak, and therefore close at hand, his hands eluding him, so to speak, at the moment of tying this knot; that is, of knotting it.
In this knotting, which he saw being done, something eluded him.
Furthermore, one clearly understands the meaning of *nouer*—both 'to knot' and 'to concoct' in French—when it's not limited to the thread, the lace, or the rope; *nouer* is whatever comes to ONE's mind.
Was it then a refusal by this kid who had grown up?
It was knotting *itself* that wasn't done, that wasn't able to be done.
But is this to say that a knot would or would not have a self—which, being there, would tie *itself*, and not being there, would leave the knotting forever unfinished?
And I had understood those who say that one knows what a knot is; even the dictionary knows; it says so in the last line of the paragraph on the meaning of the French word

for a knot, *un nœud*; it says—the dictionary does—'glans' and cites an example: – *tête de nœud*, 'dick head'. It tells us this is an insult.
That said, I have never paid real attention to popular interpretations.
I say—to the image taker—that this nonsense matters little to me; what the hands aren't able to do is to knot; hence the title of the film: – *Le Moindre geste* (*The Slightest Gesture*). . . .What's implied: it's not as simple as it looks. It's a masterpiece.
As for the IMAGEs—to return to the level of our anchor—it's faulty; it's lacking, and this is why the knot can't tie itself, or be tied—it matters little which.
And it's a question of IMAGEs and not language as claimed by those for whom the child is only a being of language.
That said, it was a question of another film, not the one in preparation among us, and the kid—the one in the photo—knows how to tie a knot, and his hands are capable of many other things that would surprise us if we could attend the gala: what the hands of a kid from the favelas are capable of doing, even if the kid is only nine or ten, as this one is.
And the rope still proves rich in IMAGEs. Everything that ONE can do with a rope—ONE being the Man-that-we-are—is there, germinating, from hanging one's contemporaries, as Traven recounts in *The Rebellion of the Hanged*, to helping one of these same contemporaries, who's crashing into the mountain fifty metres below. And the little Brazilian knew the rope's ancestor—its natural ancestor, the vine; because of his place of origin, the little Brazilian is close to the jungle down in the Amazon where those of us lived who created, as it were, the first raft, the ancestral raft, which was held together by vine rather than rope, but is otherwise the same as the one we see in the photo.
That said, the little kid is just as much from Italy, or Spain, or who knows where in Africa, as he is from Brazil; his origins lie there and perhaps also among the indigenous of the Amazon. Make a raft? The image came to him, from who knows where. . . .

*
* *

I wouldn't dream of the idea that HE has it in his blood—as ONE says.
When HE is a beaver, he can easily build a dam and a lodge, even though during his life, HE has never seen another beaver at work.
ONE is surprised, but only just.
Yet it's understood that the Man that we are doesn't know how to do anything—except learn.
And that says it all.

*
* *

The IMAGEs remains, and it can't be learnt.

*

* *

What can't be learnt or taken.[7]
Is it found?
The IMAGEs is the real find.

*

* *

It could be that the Man-that-we-are has as many memories as a camel has stomachs. And another is made here: The camera is memory, in other words, a cemetery of IMAGEs.

*

* *

Our friend WITT. once wrote:
– 'What the picture tells me is itself.'[8, 9]
Even if it means:
– 'For reality, explaining itself in language is already a detour.'
Here one sees that the image is a scapegoat; it's the image that does the saying, and reality is explained.
It was time to put the word out of use; it's the word's fault that ONE doesn't know what it says anymore.

*

* *

For as long as the image is assumed to do the saying—even if it's only in the writings of a famous philosopher—we won't be out of the woods 'Of good language.'

*

* *

'Language is a detour,' says one, and the other:
– 'It may be that language is only a mode of distended relation.'[10]
Is the IMAGEs more direct?

The IMAGEs is not language, and if ONE attempts to take it as a form of relation—among one another—there will be damage to the Institutions—which are masterpieces of language.

*
* *

If language is a detour, is the image a shortcut?
A shortcut to what?
Does the image put one and the other in direct relation? Without language, there is no other and no one.
ONE would be lost without 'I', or 'you', or 'she', or 'he'.

*
* *

Is IMAGEs a find—*une trouvaille*?
It's true that the French word stirs us, resonating rather joyously, whereas a 'discovery', *une découverte*, doesn't cause us to jump for joy.
Trouvaille . . . the word feels, based on the sound of it, like *sonnailles*, jingle bells.
– 'I've made some finds'—'*J'ai fait trouvailles*'—and the bells ring out.

*
* *

We understand that the image taker is on the lookout; if the IMAGEs is a find, one need only find the way to go about making the find, *faire trouvaille*.
But is it a question of 'making', *faire*?
We say: *Il fait bon*, it's a nice day.
But what is *IL* and what has it done, *qu'a-t-IL fait*?

*
* *

Faire is a verb that I fear.
After living close to autistic beings for a long while, it's become clear to me that wanting to make them do something—*vouloir leur faire faire*—is torture—and just as much for one as for the other, if in fact there is one and the other.
Some believe that torture is the best method. Torture has been around for a good long time. Even in its most degraded form, I avoid having to use it.

So: – Making the find, *faire trouvaille*?
I prefer acting over doing.[11]
– It's a question of IMAGEs.

*
* *

In every person, there is a sleeping tyrant. . . .
This is well known.
In every person there is a sleeping slave. . . .
And this is also true. . . .

*
* *

It's a question of IMAGEs . . . and it's a find. It's a question then of acting, *il s'agit d'agir*, rather than doing.
Alas, we only know how to do.
In my language, doing involves intention, whereas acting can surprise.
The IMAGEs surprises.
And yet acting demands care, precautions, and rigour—so much so that in practice we realise that compared to acting, doing—doing anything—is a joke.
An IMAGEs that appears without surprising will be any old thing—except IMAGEs.

*
* *

We must increase the rigour, distrust the abuses of language—language is quick to say, above all when what it says is nonsense, which it repeats—and refrain from . . . and from . . . and the IMAGEs appears. . . .
And from where and how, ONE will never know.

*
* *

Barthes said about photographs:

– 'For a photograph to be—to make—IMAGEs, at a certain point, there must be something that ONE didn't see—at the moment of taking—(therefore didn't *want* to take.)'[12]

And, once the photo is printed, it's all ONE can see. . . .
He said this in his words, but if I translate them, I don't think I'm forcing it.

*
* *

There may be times when the IMAGEs passes, fleetingly, in the eye of the image taker.
He glimpsed it. . . .
Or in the very moment when the camera was rolling, he sort of sensed it because of a premonition; the IMAGEs is event.

*
* *

If premonitory had a verb, it would be the verb for the image taker to put into practice. *Trouveur*, 'finder', one could say. *Troveor*, 'troubadour', was commonly used in the twelfth century; it was the author, the person who finds, invents. Who knows if it's a question of finding or inventing.

*
* *

With the vocabulary all broken up, the image taker is keen on passing through here.
He tells me it suits him.
Likewise, when he has back trouble, he goes to see an osteopath.

*
* *

Language without intention doesn't hold up well.

*
* *

Acting—in my language—is not a product of intention, but of IMAGEs.
This is why our friend WITT. tangles image and intention.
He was—as I have been—a teacher in classes where most of the children were slow; in his classes, there were no autistic children; what a pity.
He had students at Cambridge.

Although he never managed to untangle acting from doing, he would have experienced—witnessed first-hand—the human being in the vacancy of language, and he would not have written:

– 'The picture was supposed to be the most direct language.'[13]

He would not have saddled the image with language, in any shape or form.

*

* *

– '"Language" is only languages. . . .Languages *are* systems.'

Thus speaks he—he being our friend WITT.

I would add—if I dared:

– 'Languages belong to one mode of thinking.'

But who knows if this mode of thinking has languages or if these languages have a mode of [thinking].

It matters little—and with good reason; the person who will decide has not been born yet.

And the IMAGEs is a different mode of thinking—that which has IMAGEs; or rather, it's IMAGEs that is, or has, a whole mode of thinking.

*

* *

– 'I read a story and don't give a hang about any system of language. I simply read, have impressions, see pictures in my mind's eye, etc. I make the story pass before me like pictures . . . '

My word, our friend WITT. thinks he's in the cinema, where 'that' passes on the screen.

But he's far from certain 'that' which passes before him is the image—in my language.

The occasional cineaste has made a film with 'that'.

They would have been better off going fishing for frogs.

*

* *

It would be enough to agree on the meaning of words. . . .

Or to expect hens to have teeth.

*

* *

The image is utopian. . . .
It could be that the IMAGEs doesn't take place.
Which doesn't mean that it doesn't exist.
Who's to say what the place of life is?

*
* *

Where does life take place?
Where the IMAGEs takes place . . .
As for language, it takes place in itself.
This is why we don't leave it.
I have proposed that the IMAGEs be placed outside in order to attempt to leave it—'it' being language. . . .
Just like the crew of a ship that has run aground and casts an anchor in the distance to haul it out of there—if possible.
Parler d'image? When talking about the image, we must decide that rather than 'about', the '*d*' means '*d'où*', 'where', and then get to it, get there; and if not get to it, grab hold of it.

*
* *

And if films were IMAGEs—even if only in some small way—just anchors wet here and there to attempt to pull us out of IT—IT being what everyone would like to get out of if they could . . .

*
* *

And to say that IMAGEs is within reach, and not only say it, but act it.

*
* *

The image can be literal.
Whereas language can only be figurative.

*
* *

The three autistic kids—who are growing up—are on bread—as we say. . . .
Sometimes they give us a helping hand. Before the dough goes to the oven, it's placed on trays the kids carry from one spot to another. The trays have to be handled with great concern for horizontality.
One of us puts a glass full of water on a tray, and the tray is carried exactly as it should be.
And yet, a glass of water doesn't mean anything.

*
* *

And what do the Chinese jugglers in the Beijing Circus mean?
There is a crowd.
To see them 'do'?
To see them act.
The glasses of water in their number are their affair—what their a-act is can't be said.

*
* *

If, as I think it does, the IMAGEs ricochets off the memory of the species, whoever perceives it—the IMAGEs—will not be confused.
The IMAGEs will be interpreted in less than the blink of an eye. And whoever has perceived it—the IMAGEs—perceived it and interpreted it, will be quite proud to—finally—have something else to do other than swallow as best they can what ONE has prepared for them.

*
* *

If the IMAGEs ricochets off the memory of the species, we should not be surprised that it doesn't draw from the—symbolic—depths.

I ask *myself* what words mean—what they want to say.
Because, who can one ask?
And, that said, I ask *myself* WHO put them in charge of this wanting—to say, it seems?

*
* *

The IMAGEs ricochets off the memory of the species.
Better to say 'on'; the IMAGEs ricochets *on* this strange memory, just like—flat—pebbles thrown obliquely on the surface of water.
Which avoids locating the source of the IMAGEs in who knows what hidden recess of the heart.
We'll say: The IMAGEs is found by ricochet.

*
* *

The image taker is all pensive: He must be wondering—in his head—how he's going to go about making anything ricochet on his eye—which is a camera.
In the same way, our brains are very close to our eyes—you could say they're in our eyes—or nearly so. But then our brains are also in our hands; there is a little bit of them in all our organs. These brains of ours are therefore close to our eyes, just like the film, behind the lens, is on the lookout.

*
* *

Premonition, I said to the image taker looking out for ricochets.
One could also say acuity, because acuity grows sharper with practice, acuity that speaks of *acute* and *intense* and above all the *finesse* of discriminative sensitivity.

*
* *

I say to the image taker:

- 'Think of the sun and its myriad reflections—which people say ricochet. . . .
- That said, don't go looking at the sun; your cornea will suffer so much that you'll be forced to become a sound taker.
- In looking at the IMAGEs, you're not risking much; you'll see nothing, the absolute Nothing. I'm unaware of any damage that could be caused by all that time spent contemplating the Nothing in the frame and elsewhere. That's what they say, the frame, when talking cinema.'

*
* *

I recommend that the image taker—and everyone else—get hold, without delay, of those short works whose authors celebrate language.
Language loses its gravity in these short works.
Put otherwise, they prevent us—a little bit—from gravitating to—which is obeying—language.
And of course the memory of the species is not fertile when it comes to freedom.
But if we mix the two?

*
* *

Hermann's tortoise—the most common species of tortoise—has existed for at least 250 million years. And yet, during all this time, there have been cataclysms that annihilated living species—or nearly so.
Hermann's tortoise was thus in the 'nearly so'.

*
* *

What does our friend WITT. tell us?
– 'Without the—linguistic—system, the linking of words is dead. . . .'
One might think that only the image has a soul. . . .
Well here we have another . . .
We'll have to come back to this one.

*
* *

The imaginary—in referring to the dictionary—has nothing to do with the IMAGEs.
Imaginary—according to the dictionary:
– 'That which only exists in the imagination, unreal, fictitious . . . '
The fact is that language is only fictitious, while the IMAGEs' ricochet is real.

*
* *

What does the dictionary say?
– 'The image is a pure creation of the spirit. . . .'
And language?

*
* *

Thus only the image would have a soul.
It's our friend WITT. who proposes this.
What do I have to say about it?
What does Hugo—Victor—say?

– 'The human body hides our reality, the reality is the soul.'[14]

And Pascal?

– 'We are made up of two opposing natures, soul and body.'[15]

Our friend WITT. clears the field; of the body, there remains the image—it alone has a soul.
When I was thirty, I would have flaunted this idea by saying:

– 'But why do they—those who believe—have to believe precisely in what doesn't exist.'

As far as I'm concerned, human beings, who are full of 'fear', can only believe.
Believing—in one thing—is to take it as real.
'Real' should thus not be the thing. Otherwise believing will be lost; only fear will remain; the Man-that-we-are will lose the taste for existence.

*
* *

Contrary to language, the IMAGEs proposes nothing.

*
* *

The IMAGEs has no meaning.
That said, at any moment, it can be full of it.
ONE need only see it.

*
* *

What does our friend WITT. say?

– 'One can imagine a man inventing language, imagine him discovering how to train other human beings to work in his place, training them through reward and punishment to perform certain tasks when he shouts. This discovery would be like the invention of a machine.'

*
* *

In reading our friend WITT.—among others—evidence appears that language is understood just like the iceberg is seen.
What is perceived of language is the part of the iceberg that emerges from the water, about one-eighth.
There remains what is not perceived, this remaining part being tacit, which is why it's not said.
Would this be image? It could be. I can't say it any better.

*
* *

Nonetheless, if I believe our friend WITT., the image could have a soul—and would be alone in having one, if so.
I would not have given this any thought, as I'm not particularly preoccupied by the soul and what it can be, and who has one, and who doesn't.
But our friend WITT. thinks about this. He doesn't speak lightly; he has a hell of an Irish mug even though he was born in Austria. So much so that he makes ethics into a singular idea, defining it as the 'desire that drives us'—no doubt in the back—'to run against the boundaries of language'.
Which leads ONE to wonder if he might be a bit mystical. . . .Hence the soul with which the image would be provided—to the detriment of the rest of creation.
But the image is very different from the everyperson. It's a whole world.
And it's therefore this world that would have a soul—while the world of language would not.

*
* *

If the image—as I understand it—is that without which animals of the same species would not agree, this world would have a soul, while we would be lacking—we, the Man-that-we-are.
This proposal delights me; it gets people back on their feet; it's about time.
If this remark were democratically put to the vote, the Algonquins would already be in favour.

*
* *

It matters little to me whether I have *une âme*—whether I have a soul or not—if I don't even know what *âme* means; having read the dictionary, what's clear to me is that *l'âme* is also the bore of a firearm.

What do I have in common with a firearm?

*
* *

What does renowned ethnologist Pierre Clastres say?

– 'The woman frees the child from the earth, the man liberates him from his mother. Text and image, the myth of origin and the ritual of birth express and illustrate one another, and every time a child is born, the Guayaki unconsciously repeat the first episode in Guayaki history in a gesture which must be read in the same way that one listens to a spoken word.'[16]

P. Clastres describes what he witnessed: The newborn child is still on the ground, between the mother's legs; a man cuts the umbilical cord, meticulously cleans the child, and hands it to a woman who hoists it up:

– 'To be born in the sense of falling is, so to speak, not yet to be born, and the act of lifting assures the infant access to, ascension to, human existence. . . .'

I understand this well—and I understand, in passing, P. Clastres's predilection for that which liberates.

But what would he say if he had witnessed the birth of a bear cub?

What to say then, when the gesture is no longer 'read in the same way that one listens to a spoken word'?

Would the bear's gestures and—more generally—everything that is acted be strictly useful?

This is not the case, and ONE knows it.

So what can ONE say about the space between any gesture made and the strictly essential?

Could this—undeniable—space be due to the IMAGEs? This should come as no surprise.

*
* *

IF the image—which I speak about while knowing that language can do nothing, not help understand it, nor describe it—is alone possessed of a soul—and how not to trust the words of a philosopher who has taught at Cambridge—we can see that the image taker has an unprecedented task.

It's up to him to discover, by means of the image, what little soul still remains in this world.

*
* *

Just as the Guayaki hunter is equipped with a bow and arrows, the hunter of images has the camera—and, I hope, has got it well in hand.
He's going to hunt the soul of this land of ours, and not hunt it out, but quite the contrary, hunt it in—just as the Guayaki do with the prey they catch.

*
* *

But what does he capture with his camera?
Is it really an image; or any old thing?
Who will decide?
The everyperson who sees what's been captured.
If it's an image, they'll be delighted.

*
* *

Movement can be recreated; it's just watching image after image.
But why talk about image when shots are involved, shots taken one after the other and, between each shot taken, ONE moves things in such a way that movement is born; it comes from the eye of the watcher, the eye and the brain that is not far away.
It could be that image only appears because of a subterfuge. . . .
But which one?

*
* *

Go on then and untangle the HE from the ONE.
HE tells me.

But it won't be ONE who speaks through the mediating vocal cords of the HE who tells me—who tells me what ONE says.
And i—of individuals, that is—what do they say?
What is i's part, and ONE's, in what HE tells me—or what I tell myself?

*
* *

And who will untangle the i—of image—from the S, which could be the great Self,[17] but which is, in this case, the symbolic?

*

* *

There are those who believe that the hour is the hour.
But it isn't, not at all; it's a way of understanding.

*

* *

Where did ONE find out that there is someone—or someone else—anywhere in this existence of ours?

*

* *

Expressing oneself is part of the programme—at school, on the radio, in cinema-television, and in literature.
And it's true; the Self is part of the programme.
It remains to be seen what it is elsewhere.

*

* *

On a beautiful 14 July morning, there would be nobody on the Champs-Élysées—nobody, I mean, not even a mouse; not even a mouse—except the army parading.[18]
Impossible, you say? Of course; except in cinema.
And if cinema, whether big screen or small, asked *itself* what's good to take and what's good to leave—out of frame . . .
Itself . . . ?
But who do you expect cinema-television to ask.

*

* *

I'm less and less certain—age plays a part—that the various tricks ONE crams into our eyes and ears hold any more of an attraction than did water insects and newts moving around in moats when I was ten.

*

* *

On a page written some years ago, I find:

– 'The IMAGEs is to the work of art what chance is to the dice game.'

Because chance is a dice game. The word *hasard*, chance, comes to us from Arabia after being crossed with Spanish along the way.

The dice game is therefore chance itself; better yet, it's what appears on each of the faces of the three dice and is counted in points, and it's chance when the point that has appeared wins because of an entirely arbitrary rule that has decided it thus—that three points, that is, the ace on each face, is worth seven chips.

Chance is therefore lucky.

*

* *

Our friend WITT. tells us:

– 'Whereof one cannot speak, thereof one must be silent.'[19]

But have we ever seen ONE keep silent?

ONE speaks (about) everything.

Hence ONE tells oneself that everything is language.

*

* *

According to our friend WITT., in a sense, the image is the very bone of intention.

And we know the extent to which a bone can be devoid of intention.

*

* *

And, before the dice that decided on the word *hasard*?

Before the dice, the gods no doubt; the gods who are not devoid of intentions.

*

* *

We must thus choose—if only so we know what to expect: Who rules the world, dice or gods?
Some people—no doubt most—will say: a bit of both, so you don't fall out with one or the other.

*
* *

I imagine someone who plays dice to roll them—and nothing else, and not the other way round—someone who deeply loves the sound of the little carved bones spinning on the wooden table.
The dots marked on the faces matter little to this person; yet they continue, if only to hide the fact that they're not playing, but rolling the dice, for no reason, with no intention.
Is this acting humanly?
I think so.
But one way or another, ONE is going to take care of them—and make them speak.
The ethnologist P. Clastres tells us so. He speaks of the Atchei and their savagery as being:

– '. . . formed of silence; it was a distressing sign of their last freedom, and I too [me, the ethnologist] wanted to deprive them of it. I had to bargain with death . . . '

Is silence thus synonymous with death?

– '. . . with patience and cunning, using a little bribery (offers of presents and food, all sorts of friendly gestures, and gentle, even unctuous language), I had to break through the Strangers' passive resistance, interfere with their freedom, and make them talk. . . .'

Surprising passage: The ethnologist—a staunch libertarian—makes his confession. A few pages on, P. Clastres writes:

– 'The obligation to use the instrument of non-coercion—language—*every time it is necessary*.'

Language considered as an instrument of non-coercion is worth a detour, even if it's to the land of the Atchei, who live, I believe, in the darkest depths of Paraguay.
The ethnologist found what he was looking for there, an easy-going form of State where all the leader did was talk.
And what does this leader say—he who commands nothing sufficient to maintain the State—or Power, whichever one likes.

*
* *

The Atchei remain silent before our man the ethnologist.
Ultimate freedom, he says; but it's the need-to-speak that wins out—for this freedom, to remain silent is death.
The death of what?

*
* *

Perhaps the death of all freedom?
This should come as no surprise.
Ultimate freedom, silence.
This silence being the death—in the short term—of this very freedom.
But perhaps they experience another form of it—of freedom?
Could we live without speaking? Us?
Well . . . being the Man-that-we-are, we are mankind—like all peoples, no matter how small—who speak to each other.
And it will be necessary for people to take advantage of this freedom-of-ours.
And to be necessary, *falloir*—if we go back to the origin of the word—means to be wrong: it comes from the word *faillir*, to fail.
We can't leave—language.
This is why I suggest we resort to the image.

*
* *

Let us imagine a State where the citizens have complete freedom to speak.
Would they therefore be free?
They would have complete freedom. . . .
But freedom is not just something you have.
You still have to be—free.

*
* *

Language appears to have some sacred aspect to it.
Those that haven't got it had it—and lost it; they're now deprived of it.
So they say about agriculture, agriculture and property.
At some point, one should read what Darwin, the great Darwin, writes about a tribe in Tierra del Fuego that doesn't have—that doesn't even have—a sense of property.
These beings have nothing.
And so, Darwin says, they will be nothing, forever.

It's that simple.
It's necessary to have—even if it's only language, which is truly the least of things.

*
* *

What would the human being be without language?
They would be another being, quite simply.

*
* *

The image taker who plays with the symbolic has the wrong instrument.
In having the wrong instrument, he deceives whoever hears/sees his work.
And significantly.

*
* *

If the opportunity for language was voted on in a referendum across the cities of the world, there is no doubt that it would receive ninety-three per cent of the vote.
And with good reason; the image says nothing, to anyone more primitive than the most 'backwards' people on the globe.

*
* *

Language can undoubtedly be voted on. It's a tyrant with a good reputation. We sometimes speak about the power of words.
Like the tyrant, language only ever has the power that is given to it—by its subjects.
Certainly and without doubt, language can say: it can say that it exists, it can also say that one has to say.
But who decrees what's mandatory? The ministers of religion, whoever they are.

*
* *

To know, the dictionary says, is to be able to affirm the existence of . . .

*
* *

Refusal—whether he's conscious of it or not, P. Clastres speaks of a sociological refusal that would thus be unconscious—and thus intervenes immediately when it comes to silence.
There is no such thing as having nothing to say.
Anyone who doesn't have language is—immediately—assumed to have refused it.
Refusal always takes the blame; it denounces intention—which is therefore a culprit in the case of refusal.

*
* *

Anyone who obstinately keeps their silence seriously attacks the freedom of speech. Because being able to speak is freedom, and freedom is obligatory; it demands, it seems, that everyone speak. In the communication system, silence is like a bubble of air in the blood, lethal.

*
* *

If someone demands silence, it's not for their sake; it's to hear.
And silence is not heard.
Yet in this silence, what unfolds is that which allows the slightest word to be heard—understood.

*
* *

When I was a teacher, I occasionally had silence reign in my small class, something I was quite proud of, especially since I worked without coercion.
Now, it seems the noise of language must reign, even if it means forcing to speak those who would prefer to keep silent.

*
* *

Silence is not the absence of noise; it's noise that is the absence of silence.
In any dictionary, silence is: the fact of not . . . speaking, it's also the attitude of a person who doesn't . . . speak.
You could say that silence only exists because of the fact of *not*—more particularly, not speaking.

*
* *

Silence imposes itself—on the surface or by weight?

*
* *

Silence is made . . . which is even more extraordinary; silence is made, like crêpes.
But with what? I haven't got a clue what silence is made with, but I can say how I obtained it in my class.
I would listen very attentively, very visibly, to a clock face hanging on the wall; nothing but the face, to learn the Roman numerals.
The kids listened . . .
There was silence.
I was filled with wonder; the kids were too; they had never heard that silence.

*
* *

The Man-that-we-are is afraid of silence, just like the Guayaki were afraid of becoming animals again, and so shaved scrupulously.

*
* *

At one psychiatric institution, I established myself as the keeper of a greenhouse where anyone who wanted to could go and paint. I never would have guessed that so many mentally ill people wished to paint.
It's because painting was a decoy; in that greenhouse, ONE—everyone—had the absolute right to keep silent.

*
* *

Silence is misunderstood.

*
* *

Language?
Like *les aiguilles*, the hands, are to the clock.
And what happens is that *les aiguilles*, the needles, start to knit.

*
* *

Language is learnt.
Always already there, the IMAGEs is not learnt—nor is it taken.

*
* *

Language doesn't allow us to evoke IMAGEs.
It's not made for that.
It's made to free us from IMAGEs.
This is why the most sensible ethnologist feels responsible—perhaps without knowing it—for exporting the use of language.[20] That said, the most savage tribes, that are the furthest from us, the most 'backwards', have had language for a good long time, and practise it with a remarkable ability.

*
* *

– 'If they don't say a word, it's because they keep silent . . . '
This trivial evidence is, in fact, the most twisted of all evidence that has appeared to the Man-that-we-are.
On the basis of it, everything happens as if everyone had the right to make the other speak—and not only the right, but the imperious duty.
And so, 'patience and cunning . . . a little bribery . . . offers of presents . . . all sorts of friendly gestures, and gentle, even unctuous language . . . to break through the Strangers' passive resistance, interfere with their freedom, and make them talk.' Thus speaks the most advanced ethnologist.

*
* *

If I were an ethnologist, I would settle down here or there, without giving it too much thought ahead of time, trusting chance just as much as my projects; and, having settled close to a water source, in the shade, I would give myself up, with a happy heart, to whatever work my hands felt attracted to.
And one day or another, some individuals from some tribe—any which one—would come and see me from up close. If talking to me meant nothing to them, I would have nothing to say.

*
* *

Once upon a time there was a tribe that ONE confined to a reservation that had been established for them.
They became mute.

Rather than making one or another of this tribe speak, it would be better to return the stolen paths.

*
* *

Engaging in the study of the IMAGEs has nothing to do with some 'logy'.
ONE is going to have to get used to this.

*
* *

IMAGEs, that which ricochets off the memory of the species in all beings, whether they be human.

*
* *

Someone looks at a landscape, and says:
– 'This says something to me . . . '
Here one sees that the landscape is less reticent than those 'natives' who, stubbornly, don't speak.

*
* *

– 'This says something to me . . . '
Instead of saying:
– 'This reminds me, more or less vaguely, that this is déjà-vu.'
Here one understands that the detour is through the memory of education . . .
While the Aborigines who roam the red deserts of Australia in search of a water source seem capable of detecting the slightest detail in the landscape at a glance.
There are thus at least two memories: a reflected memory and an immediate memory.

*
* *

As soon as freedom—as ONE says—exposes itself, it's on the brink of withering.

*
* *

The subject has no choice but to express themself . . . even if it's to the detriment of the IMAGEs.

*
* *

It would be enough to listen closely to a word like 'subject'—only it would need to be amplified ten thousand times, amplified for the ear. All that swarms about in there . . .

*
* *

– 'Thus they'—the emigrants in *The Grapes of Wrath*—'changed their social life—changed as in the whole universe only man can change.'[21]
Thus speaks the Nobel Prize winner, and what he says is a blunder, a blunder like a bumblebee that buzzes as it browses for nectar, and like the buzzing of a thousand or ten thousand voices, or the drone of bagpipes over the centuries.
And this bumblebee flies around the heights of the highest institutions.
Those who preach thus—that it's only Man in the universe—no doubt believe they're uttering an enlightened truth, while they plunge their fellow beings a little further into an appalling solitude that makes them capable of any whim, including that of annihilating our fellow beings, themselves, and the rest along with them.

*
* *

Ethics . . .
The enthusiastic and desperate desire that causes us to trip and stumble over language, which is only able to say what it can say, and creates a world with nothing human in it—no matter what ONE says.

*
* *

ONE is without a doubt Man, Man saying to himself.
What I write here is written in the dictionary.

*
* *

The other day, the image taker told me that after a recent shoot—one in which he was both a character and another of those behind the camera—he looked down and saw a huge fossil in the rough grass. He had known full well he was going to find the fossil, as he himself had put it there moments prior, and when he did, a project came to him, all by itself, so to speak: He would look to the sky, wondering where it had fallen from, this large fossil whose imprint was nestled in a large stone.
And he repeated that this came to him quite by itself, *this* being the project that entailed a gesture—that of raising his head—and thus a progest, so to speak.
He didn't say the word progest; it's the present writer's find.
This progest deserves to be talked about, as it's where the detour by way of the planned project is cut out.
But can a gesture be made without a project, that is, without intention?
So it is with a reflex.
Gester, to gesture, doesn't exist in French; one must go as far as 'gestation', and not stop prior.
The word progest would cut short the detour by way of the gestation—of the slightest gesture.
If this progest has no—is not—intention, it could be IMAGEs.
But then in this case, raising one's head to the sky is to be befallen by bad luck, or to put it better, ill-timing.
Because there is no doubt that this gesture speaks; it says: – Where did that fall from?
And this progest is no longer a progest, as it's an attitude, and a deliberate attitude, even if it's deep inside the character's heart.

*
* *

When speaking of cinema, there is no way to escape the ever-present heart.
Just like the ONE who sees everything, hears everything, the heart is there, and as ONE wants to make us hear and believe, it's stuffed full of mortal anguish and sexuality, which constantly chomp at the bit, and recur.
And this is delicious jam to spread on the film, relentlessly; it's the good stuff, and the only stuff, perpetually. The film has to be chewed over and cooked up, the juice has to overflow; overflow, there can never be enough of it.

*
* *

What is it all about, exactly, speaking of IMAGEs, giving camering a shot?
It's about breaking the spell, *l'envoûtement*, of the sign.
And the dictionary tells me that '*voûte*', was *vout* in Old French, which means face, and image.

*
* *

To give a good analogy, seeing a word elude language has got to be as rare as seeing a pebble elude the earth's gravitational pull.

*
* *

That said, we must persist.
The other night, the radio told us that Jesus Christ himself, no doubt a little weary of the sceptical apostles, chose a few of them to show who he was, just as he was—that is, god.
Having done this, he told these first-hand witnesses to shut their traps about what they had just seen. Surprising words.
Could there thus be—in the eyes of god—facts that elude language?

*
* *

Someone who must be a philosopher writes to me:
– 'For me, the act is not a fact.'
Having, for my part, read and reread our friend WITT., I guessed what he was getting at, the 'who' being tacit.
The philosopher is thus right—so to speak—if we expect the fact to be language.

When I speak about acting—as I do—acting then is not language.
If it's not language, could it be IMAGEs?
It could be.
Hence my point:
– 'There are facts—of language—and there are facts of IMAGEs, the same fact being of both.'

*
* *

Is the world the same if ONE sees it from here—below—and if ONE sees it from the moon?

*
* *

The fact is . . . that etc. . . .
ONE says this, constantly.
What a fact is remains to be seen.
Some would say:
– 'It's what is seen (by the self).'
Or:
– 'It's what is the case.'
Our friend WITT., a philosopher, says:[22]
– 'The world is the totality of facts . . . these being *all* the facts.'
– 'What is the case, the fact, is the existence of atomic facts.'
I say to the other philosopher:
– 'The fact is that . . . '
and they see nothing.
What to do?
Go and watch the albatrosses fly—just as our friend WITT. did. And the fact is that the albatrosses came to him.

*
* *

– 'What is the case, the fact . . . '
But where? And for whom?
What is the case for one could very well not be for the other.

*
* *

We should say:
– 'The fact addresses . . . '
A fact exists for no one in particular.

*
* *

The fact is that a fact is not (like) a pebble; it only exists when it's said—or seen—by whoever is in the position to say it.
Because:
– 'The world is the totality of facts.'
It's still necessary for facts to be said (by the self). And in this case, the *self* is everyone among us who is destined to take up language—and thus the moon that says of itself: I'm nothing but a big pebble.

*
* *

I think it's useful—even necessary—for human beings to exercise—as soon as possible, as soon as they can speak—the power of language.
Example exercise; say to the child:
– 'You can say anything . . . '
And say to them:
– 'But you can clearly see that this doesn't mean a thing until you know what anything entails.'

*
* *

To say anything . . .
And if no one ever says anything to them, it's the end of the world.
There remains the one who (has) said.
That's god; and then it all starts again, from nothingness.

*
* *

The image taker doesn't give a damn—about all that; he just doesn't give a damn, and no harm done; he's waiting for us to talk IMAGEs.
But if talking IMAGEs is to get hold of the other world—the IMAGEs-world—it's best to stay quiet.

*

* *

Our friend WITT. talks about fact; he searches for a unity of language to count on.

*

* *

A cineaste should recognise themself by the fact that they never talk about IMAGEs.

*

* *

Parler d'IMAGEs? When talking about the IMAGEs, where does the '*d'*'—which the dictionary tells us denotes a specific origin or belonging—come from?
If rather than 'about', the '*d'*' means '*d'où*', 'where', where is the IMAGEs from?
And if this '*d'*' denotes belonging, we still need to know to what or to whom.
Talking IMAGEs remains . . .
But the IMAGEs is not—and has no—language.

*

* *

– 'Their great god Namandu emerges from the shadows and invents the world. He first creates the Word, the substance common to the divine and the human. He assigns to humanity the destiny of collecting the Word, of existing in it and protecting it. . . .Society is the enjoyment of the common good that is the Word. . . .'[23]

Thus ONE talks—among the indigenous people of the Orinoco.
And elsewhere.

*

* *

– 'For a *large* class of cases of the employment of the word "meaning"—though not for *all*—this word can be explained in this way: the meaning of a word is its use in the language.'[24]

Thus talks our friend WITT., a renowned philosopher.
So then what's the point of dictionaries?
I had a mate who spent his free time riding an old bike; a long-handled net was tied to the contraption's frame; and this mate showed me an endless number of butterflies

in boxes with glass lids. If the boxes had a lid—a glass one—it was so the butterflies would be protected—and not to imprison them, for they were dead.
Thus are the words in the dictionary, deprived of meaning, as they're put there outside of their use. Because who can be made to believe that the uses of a butterfly—any butterfly—are to be put in a box?

*
* *

– 'Not *how* the world is, is the mystical, but *that* it is.'[25]
Always the same, our friend WITT.
Thus, a *fact* can be mystical.

*
* *

I propose:
– 'The fact that *it* is, is the mystical, and not how *it* is, but that *it* is.'
To such an extent that the other philosopher can write to tell me that in his eyes, *the act* is not a fact.
What he says is a fact—and this fact is mystical.

*
* *

That *it* is mystical—insofar as *it*—doesn't surprise me; *it* is language.
And—as we have just seen—language is mystical.

*
* *

The image I evoke—the IMAGEs—has nothing mystical about it; it doesn't show itself.

*
* *

– 'There is indeed the inexpressible. This *shows* itself; it is the mystical.'[26]
It shows itself—whatever *it* is.

And whatever *it* is, *it* conceals—evidently—a considerable part of the inexpressible.
It is thus mystical.

*
* *

The act—which is acting according to the species—is not a fact, the other philosopher says to me.
This is the philosopher who has written to me—and he's quite right.
But he says—in the same letter—that he would like to visit, to see up close those I write about, whose gestures and manners of being I say are acting.
Seeing? He'll only ever see what *he* believes.

*
* *

The king—Louis XVI—was, to our people, what the cacique is to a G… tribe down by the Orinoco.[27] He had to attend to our food.
Which he didn't do with manifest concern.
Hence the Revolution of 1789.

*
* *

All characters—in cinema—are therefore mystical—insofar as *they*.
Do *they* show themselves?
They are shown. *They* are shown in showing themselves.
But do *they* look alike? The viewer wonders.
Because viewers of this *they* make an image of them.
But is this image idea or representation?

*
* *

They—the characters—are shown in showing themselves.
The monster is not far.[28]
Yet actors are not particularly monstrous; they're not dwarves, or giants, and *they* don't weigh three hundred kilos.
So what do *they* have to show? Their talent, the talent of those who make *themselves* seen, and in showing *themselves*, what they're showing is another person.

So in this case ONE talks about identification, the psychological process through which an individual confuses what happens to another person with what happens to them, so much so that a viewer watching a film in which an actor identifies with a character simultaneously identifies with the actor and the character and with this *they* that they are—the actor who, being themself, strives to be another person whose role *they* play.
And if all that was just flan, which doesn't mean cream made of milk, eggs, and flour, but rather *wham*, that is, what blows you away, then psychology doesn't know of the IMAGEs and its attractiveness, and speaks only about the person it knows—the person with language.

*
* *

The Yanomami indigenous people have—had—the custom of mixing the ashes of the bones of their dead with mashed banana in order to take in the ashes of the deceased. Why doesn't ONE talk about this anymore?

*
* *

From Bossuet, the specialist in funeral orations:
- 'Nonsense! Does everything die, is everything buried? Does the coffin make you the animal's equal, and is there nothing in you above it?'[29]

Everything dies, except the word, and everything persists, including reiterated efforts to get *ourselves* out of it—it being the animal world.
A lot of effort and exhortation that doesn't amount to much. Whereas the Man-that-we-are learns to name animals, animals don't name us.
But apparently this is not enough. ONE is not reassured by it all.
Countless beavers with goodwill build the dam.

*
* *

Francis PONGE died—we're told—last night. I hurry to read *Le Grand Recueil* (*The Grand Collection*) and there I find written that the clay statuettes Giacometti made by hand are not only the person who 'has nothing at all left, but who has [*sic*] nothing at all . . . other than this I.'[30, 31]
PONGE sees the *I* in them—and even the *I*—as an imperious ghost whose death throes must be watched over—he says.

I see—in these statuettes—a truly original work that is image in clay; otherwise put, clay in image.
And it's this *I* that seems to me the fat with which Giacometti gets rid of the Man-that-we-are, the fat and the values.

*

* *

– 'Exhausted, thin, emaciated, naked . . . '
This is one of the statuettes, the figures made by Alberto Giacometti's hands; the figure is certainly man, and this *bonhomme*, this everyman, is emaciated to the point that if there were any less of him there would be nothing at all.
And Francis Ponge writes that this person 'who is now nothing at all'—or nearly so; who doesn't even have skin on their bones—is neither skin, nor bone; is *I*, somewhat stripped.
I'm stunned.
I—he says—is what remains—of the person—when they are and have nothing.
The everyman annihilated, *I* remains.
Stunned, I said, and stunned—*pantois*—is a word that has the same root as fantasy—*fantasme*—which ONE talks about a lot.
In this clay stretched to the point where one thinks it won't last long—and it does—Francis PONGE sees *I*, the Man—he tells Giacometti—the human Person, the free Person.
Who knows where PONGE sees freedom in this case. Via transparency? And where he gets the certainty that it's *I* he sees and not HE. He believes in *I*, no doubt; which is not enough to prove to me the existence of the *I* ONE talks about.
Admittedly, PONGE tells us where:
– 'This *I* . . . imperious ghost . . . that appears at the head of most of our sentences.'
That language can't establish itself without this ghost doesn't prove to me that the ghost exists; anyone who sees ghosts is not far from believing in the resurrection of the dead, and therefore in god. For a good long time, I was struck by the fact that the more someone thinks about not believing—in god—the more they believe in this *I* that PONGE sees—as if in the clay that has been thinned, stretched, reduced to such an extent, only the figure's attitude remains.
Is it then through attitude that *I* expresses itself and thus proves its existence?
But animals, whether wild or domesticated, don't lack attitudes. Is every animal thus a PERSON too?
ONE would think so on seeing them act.
That said, *I* being the first word in most of our sentences, we can clearly see that since animals don't use language, they have no need for this ghost, which we only see as a word.

Because it's only a matter of the word, and nothing else.
If I speak, it's clear to see that if the I was not there, what would remain is to keep quiet.
And to begin with, someone who happens to be here has told me that Giacometti's slender figures, to put it mildly, are made of bronze, not clay.
I continue to believe they're clay; one need only look at any of the 'people' who walk with a spring in their step, and who, walking at a good clip, don't advance at all. It's clear that Giacometti handled clay, and not bronze, and if the statuettes are bronze it's because they were cast in a mould, a mould left in some material—in Giacometti's clay.
Clay, *argile*, the word suits me. The figures are Alberto's clays.
If god exists, every-one-of-us resembles him, and resembles him to the point where he can't see clay that has been played with some, unless he blows inside it, or on it.
In or on, the difference is huge; either the breath brushes against it, or penetrates it.
PONGE's breath penetrates and makes a bubble, and this blown bubble is the Person; and PONGE is quite content; he said to himself that he had perhaps breathed wasted breath—into the clay, and who knows where else. He didn't waste his breath, HE became *I*, *I* finding itself in this bubble; finding itself if ONE seeks it there, and in seeking it, has one not—already—found it?

*
* *

What surprises me—dismays me?—is that I took this PONGE for the one who wrote *Le parti pris des choses* (*The Voice of Things*).[32]
Nothing but the title delighted me; it has to be said that the existence of *I* had been ringing in my ears. I have been living as close as possible to children said to be autistic—and rather close to those close to them.
Not having the use of language, would they be deprived of *I*?

*
* *

And this PONGE—who sees *I* where I only see slimmed-down clay—was, I'm told, a communist when I was one myself; and he was a responsible communist, this PONGE, while I always dodged the apparatus. Abruptly, from one day to the next, he wondered if he would be capable of sentencing someone to death—someone other than himself. Having answered, No, he considered himself disabled and thus unfit to lead. What surprised me was the time it took him to realise an obvious fact that had leapt to my eyes as the good communist that I was.
What was he going to do, this PONGE, in a leading apparatus?

In short, I liked him up until the moment that just passed, when I realised—if he's to be believed—that Giacometti's clays would be dressed up with an *I*.

*
* *

On opening the dictionary, to check—once again—what it says about this *Personne*, my eyes find—and find at once: – No human being.[33] E.g.: *Personne ne le sait.* No one knows. Having read this, my eyes turn to the etymology found at the top of the column, and it says there: – Word of Etruscan origin; – Theatre mask.
If, as PONGE assumes, Giacometti's clays are of man being burned at the stake, and thus skimmed of fat, I wonder how the Person as mask persisted through the blaze. Could the Person be made of asbestos? And who can explain to me what PONGE was going to do in the Party—the Communist Party—if he was in search of a Person—any Person at all? Instead, he finds them in anything, even Giacometti's clay—as we have just seen.

*
* *

I'm indignant, and all the more so because, without telling anyone, I had taken Giacometti as a partner, a supporter that Ponge was to erase and to erase for always, in search of what appears when everything is taken away.
Erase everything and something still remains: traces, an image.
Image of what?
And why should the image be the image of anything?
Image is image, that's all.
And here's the other, who turns up with a Person slung over their shoulder.
What is there to be offended at, as offended I am.

*
* *

When, in what era, will we find written on the walls:
– 'It is forbidden to deposit your Person here just because they're unemployed?'

*
* *

It's true that I understood nothing of this carry-on; I never understood any of it.
I have to admit that the Person is what everyone takes themself to be.
And that's all.

*

* *

– 'We must recognise the fact that the primary function of communication is to facilitate slavery.'[34]

This statement by C. Lévi-Strauss passes in silence.
Communication is one of the saints of our mode of civilisation.
Slavery? The word is surprising.
And yet, through communication, our mode of thinking becomes servile.
Barely freed from one servitude, and as if to finish off our liberation, the Man that we are rushes into another.
After the king, it's myself; after the god, the ONE, and all the 'ion' words that follow, education, preceding the others.
And it's of course a great benefit that education is compulsory.
To the detriment of what, remains to be seen.

The IMAGEs to the Detriment

If the Man-that-we-are ever came to reign on the earth as planned, ants would go to bee school from a very young age, and vice versa, and silkworms would go on training courses with spiders.

*

* *

What can pass for a joke is passé, and by far, and for a good long time now; the evil is done; irreversible. We're already a long way from the days when C. Lévi-Strauss, who later became a professor at the Collège de France, could think that if the Nambikwara roasted two or three missionaries, the latter had not earned their fate; and not only did C. Lévi-Strauss think this deep in his heart, he wrote it—in *Tristes Tropiques*—where I just read it—and no doubt reread it; I have no memory of the lines.
They invite further thought: What was C. Lévi-Strauss going to do in such a tricky situation? Realise that 'the struggle against illiteracy is indistinguishable from the increased powers exerted over the individual citizen by the central authority.'[35]
Illiterate he was not.

*

* *

That said, being able to write doesn't get you far, no further than the jobs that require the ability to do so, because now the electronic typewriter has made it necessary to respect spelling, at the risk of blowing a fuse, or who knows what part of the mechanism thanks to which one has begun to think that learning to write will soon fall into disuse. By that time, speaking our language will be as surprising as speaking Latin or Greek. And it's the machine that grumbles. The machine, not the everyman, that always agrees, regardless of what ONE makes it do.

ONE tells the everyman to kill? He goes and does it.

ONE tells the everyman to go get himself killed; the same is true and he's perhaps just as willing.

No ass has ever been this servile; even donkeys and mules have a limit that can't be passed, otherwise they lie down. Only oxen lie down to die when they can no longer toil under the yolk.

The Man-that-we-are can always go on, and if we no longer want to, another will come and outdo us.

What are we taught at school if not that we must outdo our neighbour? Why outdo? In order to outdo. It's the ABCs of competition. And so ONE tells us what place we're in. At the school I attended as a child, on Wednesdays the head teacher and principal came to our class to give us the results of the last composition: both with their bowler hats in their hands, or on the teacher's desk, and then on their heads when they left.

Thus were the elite shaped by their education—into what shape?

What do you call such learning?

And so the children of our time flourish; they have to declare their trade as soon as possible, well before they can imagine what their day-to-day life will be like if they ever get there and make it to where they said they were going. It's like a curse.

*
* *

Now is the time of the carnival barkers.

What they say didn't even make us laugh when we were thirteen. They rehash the hackneyed bawdy joke that went limp in the eighteenth century, and no doubt a long time before; that is freedom.

Freedom for whom? For speech.

*
* *

But speech is not someone who, being free, can be free or not.

Let us always begin with speech, as it's easiest.

ONE will see about the rest later.

*
* *

For Francis PONGE, as we have seen, the subject is enough.
What subject? Grammar, without which the sentence can't be formed.
But is the subject not the individual?
In our societies, what would an individual who is not a subject be? *Personne*, nobody.

*
* *

The person I call the image taker—it being understood that IMAGEs is neither taken nor seen—told me just now that only yesterday, towards late afternoon, he was waiting, his camera very much ready, for the swallows to start whirling around their nests under the eaves.
He lives in a house in the hamlet now, the white house named after the plaster covering its walls, and it's true the house stands out from the others, which have a uniform colour that can't be described; they hold earth as if they were of adobe, but what a strange adobe; dust and stones held in a wall with a bit of mortar that together make stone; and these houses stand muddled together, so that from afar they look like a troop led by a white house, and every day it's like that, the troop snug under their roofs, which are an indeterminate colour: it changes according to the light and the clouds and the season and no doubt the mood of whoever sees them from afar.
For a long time, for months and months, if not years, it has been understood that I need the swallows' nests before the species disappears, understood to such an extent that the ballet of the swallows has taken on the solidity of the tacit among us.
But then the camera jams; the repair man suggests that the image taker use another camera while we wait for him to repair the first.
The two cameras are identical; all the same, the image taker prefers to rehearse so he'll be at ease when shooting recommences.
Now he thinks about the swallows, whose nests are under the eaves overhanging the walls of the white house. So he puts his camera on battery power and waits for the swallows.
Everyone knows what happens—all too well; it only takes waiting in order for what you're waiting for not to come, and this is a constant phenomenon; every day, at all times, the white house appeared in a cloud of swallows, and now, who knows where they are.
He could capture a short sequence that would be projected under the banner of:
– 'Absence of swallows.'
It would be enough to make people believe this entailed an underground Japanese film to arouse interest among connoisseurs. The camera would have captured the

plastered walls, a window, and under the canopy of eaves, the pouches of clay lumped against the wall, the heap of pouches, and nothing else, because the swallows are not there, or in the sky, or around the stagnant puddle . . . [36]
It's no doubt a difficult matter—rather than difficult, delicate—to capture—as they say—to capture what's not there, what's lacking.
I say to him:
– 'Capture images of what's lacking.'
It could be that the images are there, in what's lacking.
And that the swallows are there; one need only see the little pouches to think of them.
Is it a question of thinking?
If so, it's thus that the cat thinks about the mouse. It's hard to believe a cat saying anything to itself; the fact is that it waits, outside the hole that's flush with the floor; it seems to have eternity to itself, and it does because if the mouse doesn't appear and the cat lying in wait dies of old age, another cat will turn up, there, to wait, and it matters little whether it's the same cat; it's the cat as a species that waits. And what do you want a species to wait for? The species waits in images; what decides the cat's presence is the image.

One sees—if one can say so—what it is about the image—the IMAGEs—that I stubbornly try to get across. Seeing a cat crouched outside a mouse hole, living entirely in its body so that, in the end, the mouse comes out, is for me proof of the existence of the IMAGEs. And so here we have the image taker, against the wall, the camera on battery power pointing at the nests. Nothing. To relax the camera a little, as he probably feels it's stiff, he goes on a brief tour of the horizon; just to see; and the camera becomes brand new; the image taker has had to be shown the surroundings, while keeping one eye on the swallows.
And it's with the other eye that he has seen an image, and it spurted into this eye: the image—because what else would you call it—of the wall studded with bullet marks that he has spent months looking everywhere for. In the film to be made, the character—whose role the image taker plays—is fascinated by these constellations, fascinated, spellbound.
Perhaps he will brush the fingertips of his left hand against the holes like a blind man, perceiving them with the flesh of his fingers; this blind man sees; what he sees, with the flesh of his fingers, is image.
For months and months, the image taker has been looking for the wall that would be his partner; you don't choose a partner lightly. And now he sees his wall in the sights of the new camera. He sees it just as he saw it, desperate not to find this wall capable of taking on its role, which is not all that simple. Because it was his teacher of times past who showed him the wall and the constellation of traces left by the bullets in the plaster, and it was Aimée who was there, standing against the wall, and he, the teacher, who was being stalked closely by militia rogues, and was wounded in the knee—a

bullet having shattered his kneecap—who was in the baker's oven, huddled up to allow Aimée to fill it with sticks as though she were about to light a fire; on hearing the militiamen running, she closed the little iron door on the teacher who they had just lost sight of. He was there, but where? To make the woman speak, they put her up against the wall, and fired again and again, lodging their bullets in the wall as knives are lodged around the body of the partner who doesn't flinch. Aimée didn't flinch. The militiamen left after ransacking the house and setting fire to it to smoke out their prey; the fire didn't catch and one of the men thought he saw a shadow in the trees. They left. Only the holes remained.

This is the story of the section of wall that the image taker has been searching for in vain, and now here it is, within camera range; it takes the eye of the camera to see it. When the image taker looks at the wall with his own eyes, the section no longer plays its role; the image taker is like the astronomer who spots a new constellation with his telescope, but then can't find it again with the naked eye.

– 'Because the eye is naked . . . '

I said this to the image taker on remembering that I had been the inhabitant of the white house. This was a long time ago, a long ten years ago, and I told him that I had leisurely contemplated this section of wall that was near the baker's oven, in the laneway, the plaster flaking, the holes that I said had been rented out by little snail fossils; this was absurd, because to reach the moment when the Hercynian chain was formed, you would have to go back hundreds of millions of years. As old as these houses may be, they're not ancient. The holes remain, in the house and the image I retain; small wonder the image taker has found it again, this lost image.

*

* *

Rather than interpreting signs, I got attached to traces.
And traces are not signs.

*

* *

The ABCs of the IMAGEs taker could be to distinguish between SIGNS and TRACES.

*

* *

Any story that respects the distinctiveness of the IMAGEs would be/make a legend.

Translated with Daniel Tunnard

Notes

1 'Le propre de l'IMAGES' was written in 1988 and first published in 2021 as part of *Camérer. À propos d'images*, Paris, L'Arachnéen, 2021.

2 Throughout the text Deligny refers to Ludwig Wittgenstein in this manner. Here he cites 'A Lecture on Ethics', which was published in *The Philosophical Review*, vol. 74, No. 1, Jan. 1965, pp. 3–12.

3 Stephen Jay Gould, *The Flamingo's Smile. Reflections in Natural History*, New York, Norton, 1985.

4 The professor in question is André Leroi-Gourhan.

5 Deligny is referring to a Moroccan child who lived close to Graniers and played the main character—a Brazilian boy—in the film project *Toits d'asile* (*Asylum Rooftops*).

6 Traven, B, *The Rebellion of the Hanged*, London, Robert Hale Limited, 1952.

7 Here Deligny plays with the paronyms *s'apprend* and *se prend*, translated as 'learnt' and 'taken'.

8 Unless otherwise stated, this and subsequent Wittgenstein quotes are from Anthony Kenny's translation of *Philosophical Grammar*, edited by Rush Rhees and published by the University of California Press in 1978.

9 In the French work, Deligny read *l'image*, which was translated by Kenny as 'the picture' rather than 'the image'.

10 Deligny cites Claude Lévi-Strauss here, and though he is likely referring to the chapter 'The Writing Lesson' of *Tristes tropiques*, the line does not appear to be a direct quotation.

11 Deligny writes that he prefers *agir*, 'acting', over *faire*, which, juxtaposed with *agir*, can be considered 'doing', though in other contexts, such as *faire trouvaille*, would more naturally be translated as 'making'.

12 Deligny is likely referencing Roland Barthes's *Camera Lucida*, not directly, in *sa langue*—Barthes's language—but rather by translating it into his own words.

13 As above and below, Kenny translated *l'image* as 'the picture' instead of 'the image'.

14 Victor Hugo, *Les Travailleurs de la mer*, Paris, Verboeckhoven, 1866.

15 Blaise Pascal, *Pensées*, Paris, Port-Royal, 1670.

16 This and subsequent quotes by Pierre Clastres are taken from Paul Auster's translation of *Chronicle of the Guayaki Indians*, published by Zone Books in 1998.

17 Rather than *Soi*, Deligny writes *Soy*, the Middle French pronoun no longer used to refer to the self.

18 Following this sentence is a fragment that could not be made out in its entirety. For the sake of coherency it has not been included in the translation.

19 Proposition 7 of Wittgenstein's *Tractatus Logico-Philosophicus*, translated by C.K. Ogden, and published by Kegan Paul, Trench, Trubner & Co., Ltd. in 1922.

20 Here Deligny alludes to Lévi-Strauss's *Tristes tropiques*.

21 John Steinbeck, *The Grapes of Wrath*, New York, Viking Press, 1939.

22 Propositions 1.1, 1.11, and 2 of *Tractatus Logico-Philosophicus*.

23 Pierre Clastres, *Archeology of Violence*, translated by Jeanine Herman, Los Angeles, Semiotext(e), 2007.

24 Section 43 of Wittgenstein's *Philosophical Investigations*, 4th edition translated by G.E.M. Anscombe, P.M.S. Hacker, and Joachim Schulte, and published by Wiley-Blackwell in 2009.

25 Proposition 6.44 of *Tractatus Logico-Philosophicus*, which references *le fait*, 'the fact', in the French translation cited by Deligny: 'Ce qui est mystique, ce n'est pas *comment* est le monde, mais *le fait* qu'il est.' (Translated by Pierre Klossowski and published by Gallimard in 1961).

26 *Ibid.*, proposition 6.522.

27 The name of the tribe is illegible.

28 The word *monstre*, 'monster', is not far from the French verb *montrer*, 'to show'.

29 *Sermons de Messire Jacques-Bénigne Bossuet, Évêque de Meaux*. . . .Tome Premier, Paris, Chez Antoine Boudet, Imprimeur du Roi, 1772.

30 This and subsequent quotes are from Ponge's essay, 'Reflections on the Statuettes, Figures, and Paintings of Alberto Giacometti' in *Le Grand recueil*, Paris, Gallimard, 1961.

31 It is not certain whether Deligny intentionally misquoted Ponge, who writes, '*L'homme non seulement n'a plus rien; mais il n'est plus rien; que ce JE.*'—'The person not only has nothing at all left, but is now nothing at all, other than this I.'

32 Francis Ponge, *The Voice of Things*, translated by Beth Archer Brombert, New York, McGraw-Hill, 1972.

33 In French, *personne* can be used as both a noun to mean an individual human being, a person, and as a pronoun to indicate either the absence of a human being, no one, or anyone.

34 Claude Lévi-Strauss, *Tristes tropiques*, translated by John Russell, London, Hutchinson, 1961.

35 *Ibid.*

36 The last word in this sentence appeared at the end of the page and was cut off.

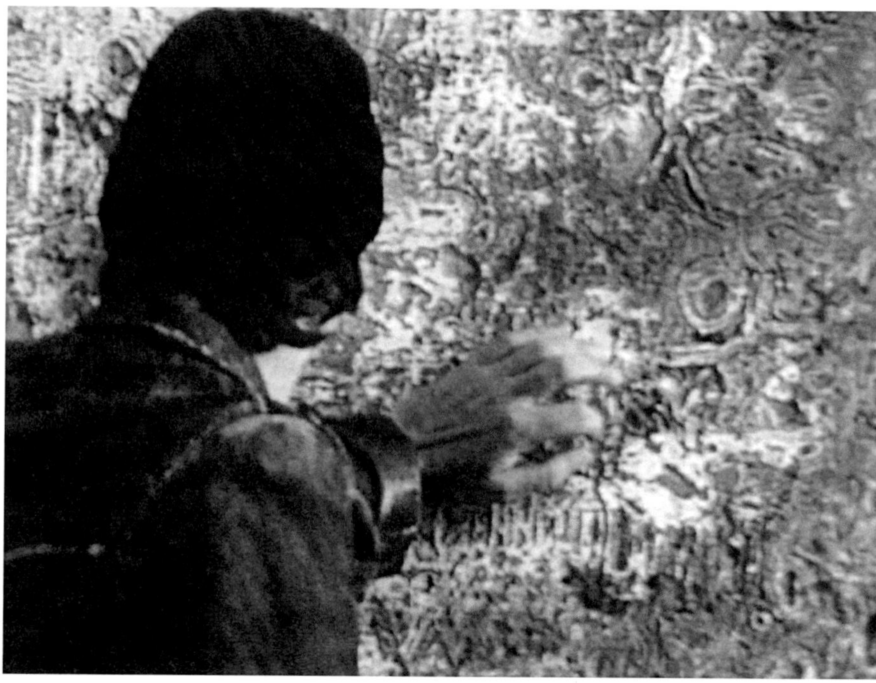

Renaud Victor in a sequence from the unfinished film *Toits d'asile* (*Asylum Rooftops*), incorporated into *Fernand Deligny. About a film to make*, 1989.

What Is Not Seen (by the Self) [1990][1]

THE ERA OF THE IMAGE. We don't live in the age of the image, regardless of what they say.

The era of the image! Even though we have never been further from the image. We're in the century of language, of chitchat, of verbalised reproduction, of unbridled speech. One has no choice but to talk. The image is what Janmari, the autistic child in *Ce Gamin, là* (*That Kid, There*), understands; it's his mode of thinking, he for whom there is no language. . . .In my life, I'm constantly grappling with this absence, this vacancy, this mode of thinking apart.

It's evident that these children, who have no use of language, think. They need to be left in peace, but the Institution can't handle that. It can't handle the absence of language, and nothing can be done about this. We need there to be language somewhere or we're lost.

People cling to the characteristic of language that preserves their singularity in relation to the animal. . . .An old fear . . .

THE IMAGE, THE ANIMAL. Now, it may be that the image is part of the animal kingdom. . . .This is no doubt very much the case: The image lies deep within the purview of the memory of the species, and the memory of the species is something that all species have in common, including the human species. . . .People can't handle that. I don't know why we can't handle the human species being taken, in the literal sense of the term, why we regard it as a species unlike the others that . . .

The image is the means by which the species persists despite everything. . . .It's a trace . . . a trace that awaits, on the lookout. . . .

This is part of what cinema entails; that is, an immediate enthusiasm. And we don't know why, but we're moved by what we end up calling images, which are not the effect of language; images move us in a way that goes well beyond language. . . .There are some who have managed this—whether they realise it or not. . . .The Tramp is one of them, of that there is no doubt: his images move us immediately, and very deeply; they overtake everyone.

There is no reason for it, no reason . . . particularly because in a work of cinema, the images are not *on* the film, so to speak; they are not inside it; they occur between the person who filmed the work and the one who watches it. It's a phenomenon that occurs 'between' and you can't master it. . . .

FREE, ON THE SCREEN. The image eludes knowledge . . . an image, if I speak my own vocabulary, is not taken. . . .
An image can't be taken; that is, be taken by the self (which is a projection of one: a different world than that of images). . . .The image is perceived, but not by the self: by a different point of view that remains more or less stricken by the perpetual collapse of the majestic *one*. . . .
. . . we can say with absolute certainty that the image takes place when the self has been evacuated. It's certain that at this moment, there is an image. . . .
Images are not taken and yet occasionally they're on the screen, and they appear on the screen as though they were delivered there. On the one hand, images are not taken; on the other, they appear as though they have been delivered; they're free, images are free; the camera is a formidable thing: The image is developed and appears, freed, on the screen.
The image taker who in the capacity of the self, s e l f, is a subject of language, is subjected to language, fatally, doesn't take the image. As long as the image taker doesn't leave the self, s, e, l, f . . . there will be no image. . . .What generally weighs on him is the weight of the self. It's the very word, the fact . . . the fact that everyone thinks they're the self.

THE WORLD OF IMAGES. This is the difference between acting and doing. When we do something it's intention, it's language: We do the prep work to make soup, we do the dishes, we do whatever you like. An autistic kid doesn't *do* anything: It's the act. This is very clear to see. This is seen by whoever has a trained eye, by whoever lives with autistic kids. The same is true of the image: In my jargon, an image is not 'made'. An image arrives, is nothing but coincidence. . . .
Now, being coincidence, the image as I understand it, the distinctiveness of the image, is autistic. I mean it doesn't talk. The image doesn't say anything! And . . . just as with autistic children, this is yet another reason for everybody to make them say whatever they like. . . .The image, too, is used as a scapegoat. . . .

A WORLD WITHOUT INTENTION. Everybody endeavours to reduce chance. The more this is the case, the more civilisation protects us, via multiple institutions, from chance . . . and what if, in a film, chance could be glimpsed? It would require 'disintentionalising', a removal of intention. . . .A film can attract folks, it can contain stories, situations, whatever comes to mind, on the condition that the attraction is nothing more than that, and provided that the image taker (for whom there remain a few after-effects from the next world) has a bit of a gift for the image. . . .They can then embark on a topic rich in images . . . perceive coincidences, be a free spirit, rid themself of all projects, and the slightest conviction. . . .

THIS IS CINEMA, IT'S WHAT IS NOT SEEN (BY THE SELF). Is *That Kid, There* a documentary or a work of fiction? It's a genuine documentary. And for good reason: You can't get Janmari to do anything other than what he does every day. One couldn't make more of a documentary than that. And it makes the film a fictional work because folks have never experienced anything like it. It's neither documentary, nor fiction; it's the customary, this customary being so real that it surprises . . . the ultra customary surprises: that is, surprise can come from what is not seen (by the self). A gesture to reach for a piece of bread can surprise if you manage 'to film' what is not seen (by the self) in the gesture, and is there in such a way that the self perceives what it would not have seen.

Why is this cinema? Because it is not seen . . . I mean reaching for a piece of bread is very common, folks do it all the time, so they perceive it tacitly, but it's not verbal expression, or doesn't end up as such.

This is cinema: It's coming to the aid of all the jerks who believe they can see, while what they see is zilch; they don't see anything. . . .The task of cinema lies here, the urgency of cinema is this: to revive that which among them is numbed, dazed, squandered, overnourished.

THE DIALOGUES OF SILENT FILM. There was silent film and then film began to speak. Images became ravaged by language: since they speak, one listens to what they say. Prior to this, they didn't 'say' anything and so cineastes were compelled to stick to what was more understated, clearer.

What's striking about our times is that in theatre, those who stand out . . . don't say anything: Samuel Beckett doesn't say anything at all and he's remarkable. What's surprising is the extent to which this marks our times. . . .Samuel Beckett is the best of a moment in time devoted to language, it's wonderful. . . .

. . . if only the dialogue in cinema was Beckett's . . .

THE IMAGE TAKER'S JOB. The verb 'to film' took just like that . . . it's always made me uncomfortable. . . .I'm well aware that what we're dealing with here is the making of a film, but how is it that the material became the verb? 'To film' is truly an infinitive that doesn't fit, and infinitives mustn't be squandered. . . .Does one say that a hen has 'egged'? Care must be taken so words don't become ill. . . .

A tool is often something that can become a verb: 'hammer', 'to hammer' . . . 'camera', 'to camer'. . . .

'Ethics' remains a nebulous word . . . like 'image', like 'asylum'. It's a word I had never used—until I read Wittgenstein. According to him, ethics is 'the desire that drives us to run against the boundaries of language'[2]. . . .Well, that's exactly what the image taker's job is, their essential job—to be impregnated with the idea of exceeding the boundaries of language and not be subjugated to whatever symbolic system you like. This is ethics.

. . . *Cahiers du Cinéma* . . . Bazin's articles . . . by chance I come across a quote by Malraux: '. . . the means of connecting the person to the world by a means other than language.' For Malraux, this is cinema. And this, too, reassured me quite a bit. . . .When it comes to my stories about images, I'm not that much of an oddball, I'm not entirely alone. . . .

As I see it, there is a tradition that was interrupted by the popularity of psychoanalysis and other modes of thinking in which language is . . . everything. . . .

. . . .And regardless of what they say, we don't live in the age of the image. . . .

Notes

1 'Ce qui ne se voit pas' is based on an interview of Deligny conducted by Serge Le Péron and Renaud Victor, who selected the material and shaped it into the piece published in *Cahiers du Cinéma*, No. 428, in February of 1990.

2 Deligny likely would have quoted Wittgenstein from the 1971 Gallimard volume *Leçons et conversations sur l'esthétique, la psychologie et la croyance religieuse suivi de Conférence sur l'éthique*, translated by Jacques Fauve. The English quote is taken from 'A Lecture on Ethics', *The Philosophical Review*, vol. 74, No. 1, Jan. 1965, pp. 3–12.

Postface
Minor Gestures, Minor Media

Elena Vogman

The architectural motif of the labyrinth appears at decisive junctures in Fernand Deligny's long essay *The Arachnean*, a text itself composed of detours, repetitions and associations of a heterogeneous nature—he draws on the fields of mythology, anthropology, philosophy and milieu theory, as well as on personal memories. It is a metaphor for endless complications followed by endless solutions: the path of Icarus on his way through the labyrinth, culminating in his tragic flight to the sun. Crucially, Deligny introduces the labyrinth as an analogy to the main figure of the text—the Arachnean, a spider's web, a network of trajectories of autistic children.

> To admit the persistence of the Arachnean would require such upheavals in the way the Man-that-we-are [*l'homme-qui-nous-sommes*] has organized themself that it is entirely reasonable to think that we will persist on the flight path that has become so ordinary and so powerful that it puts us in orbit, while hoping that what happened to Icarus won't happen to us, Icarus who was so preoccupied with escaping the detours of the labyrinth. And the Arachnean can truly be said to be rich in endless detours.[1]

According to the Greek myth, Icarus and his father Daedalus, the labyrinth's architect, are both imprisoned in the confusing structure on the island of Crete. In order to escape the labyrinth, Daedalus finds a solution—he fashions two pairs of wings out of wax and feathers for Icarus and himself. However, despite his father's warnings, Icarus cannot resist the pleasure of elevation and approaches the sun. The wax of his wings melts and he drowns in what is today the Icarian Sea.

Interestingly, the myth serves Deligny as a paradigmatic image of the mode of human behaviour, the action put in parallel with a labyrinth and Icarus's flight as a properly humanist project. In other words, Icarus's tragic fate implicitly reflects upon the condition of the 'Man-that-we-are', its finality and its teleology.

The labyrinth appears in this parallel as an obstacle, a challenge to be overcome in order to transition to the new level of the thrilling adventure where the hero once again faces his fate. Icarus rises always higher, but the myth puts an end to this 'Icarian illumination'. In opposition to this tragic end, Deligny places the Arachnean—a labyrinth without exit, which is, like a spider's web, a structure 'rich in endless detours'.

But what is an endless detour? What is its logic and its temporality? And how is one to escape the tragic finality of an action, a project, or a goal?

Here I want to explore the possibility of an 'endless detour', following Deligny's conceptualisation of the 'minor gesture' (*moindre geste*) and 'wander lines' (*lignes d'erre*). Referring to the filmic documentation of children's behaviour that gestalt psychologists Kurt Lewin and Max Wertheimer undertook in the late 1920s, my hypothesis addresses less the Icarian myth than a processual dialectics immanent in Deligny's thinking of 'endless detours'. I will argue that Deligny's idea of a 'labyrinth' implies a particular situation: a mediation of a milieu in which such detours can emerge, unfold, and, crucially, where they can be uncovered. Given this specific inscription of the milieu, the process of disclosing endless detours requires a work with an *optical unconscious*, a particular mode of constructing the gaze.

Filming Gestalt and Its Decomposition

Nowhere in his vast body of published work does Deligny mention the Berlin school of gestalt psychology's experimental film practice. Yet despite differences in their approaches and motives for observing children's behaviour, Deligny and the authors of gestalt theory had crucial elements in common. As well as their evident use of the camera for primarily non-aesthetic purposes, they shared a more fundamental aspect: the valorisation of the milieu, or 'field', of children's action.

Grounded in the assumption that the perceptual field is organised, gestalt psychologists emphasised that organisms perceive entire patterns or configurations rather than isolated elements. Human actions (*Handlungen*) are conditioned by a continuous reorganisation of the field. In order to understand the complexity of behavioural processes, Kurt Lewin and Max Wertheimer were interested in the ontogenetic development of behavioural structure. This is how in 1929 they conducted a series of experiments with their own children. They used the camera to record and examine the children's performances in the field, while defining the action as a result of what they called a framework of 'field forces' (*Feldkräfte*).

For instance, in one of their short films we see Hannah, a three-year-old girl who is given the task of sitting down on a stone. Hannah is spinning around the obstinate object, which she has placed her hands on, as if searching for support. She completes several circles, even tries to conquer the stone with her leg as though she wants to take control of it, but in vain. Lewin explains: 'In order to sit down it is first necessary to turn around and thus to make a movement contrary to the direction of the goal.' Hannah doesn't succeed in quitting the 'visual direction' and multiplies her detours. Another short film shows Hans, age seven. Without hesitation, Hans sits down straight away, briefly turning his back to the stone. According to Lewin, the reason for Hannah's failure is her inability to restructure the field. 'The action of the older child is determined by the *functional* direction rather than by the *visual* direction. The "detour" no longer constitutes a difficulty.'[2]

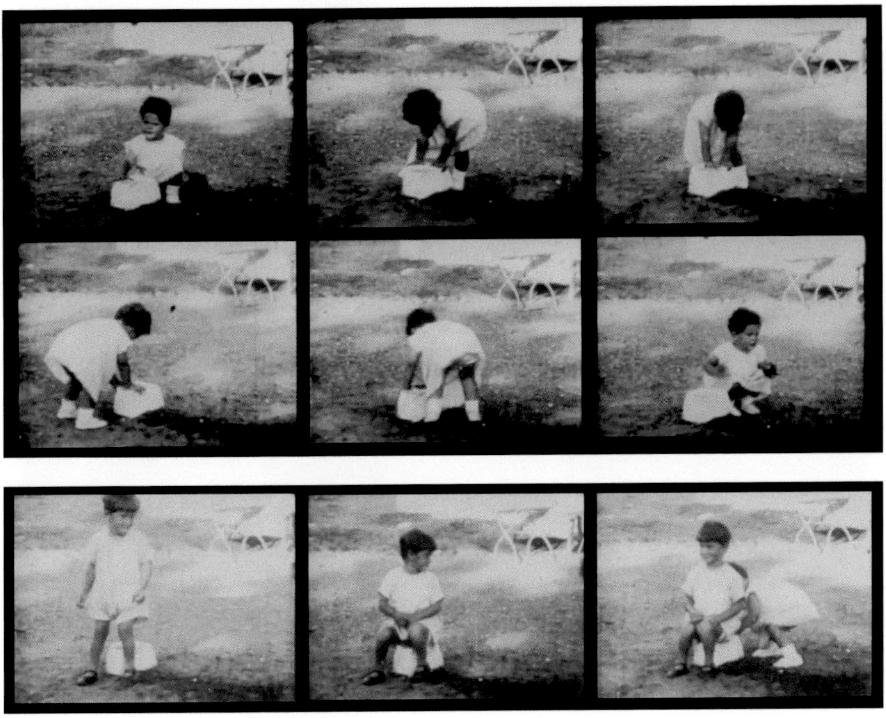

Frames from Kurt Lewin's film *Field Forces as Impediments for a Performance*, 1929.

The same year, Lewin commented on these experiments in a publication entitled *Die Entwicklung der experimentellen Willenspsychologie und die Psychotherapie (The development of experimental psychology of the will and psychotherapy)*.[3] The text contains incisive methodological arguments in favour of experimental psychology and addresses some of the critiques regarding its simplicity articulated on the side of psychoanalysis. Lewin takes an empirical and comparative approach in studying a phenomenon that Freud conceptualised as repetition compulsion (*Wiederholungszwang*). In his book, Lewin juxtaposes frames he has extracted from his films of children's actions with tracings children have made, directing his attention to the modulation of actions and gestures in time.

Tafel 3.

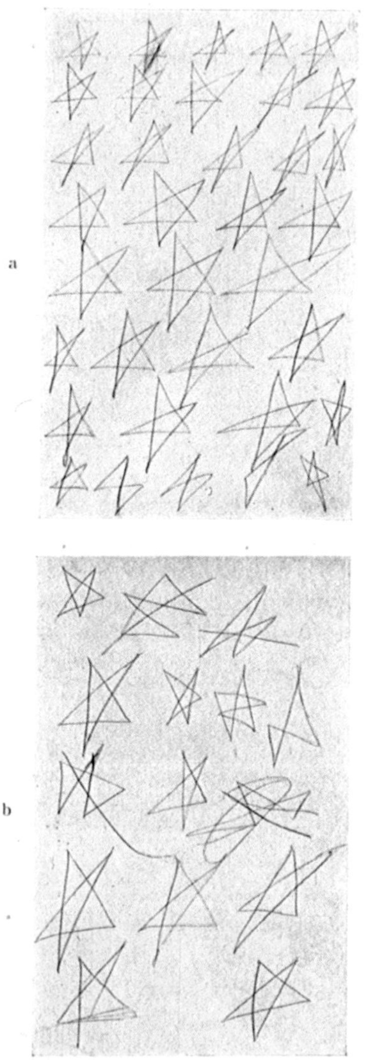

Abb. 4. Psychische Sättigung beim Pentagrammzeichnen (Kurzschluß; Gestaltzerfall; Bedeutung der Einbettung in ein größeres Ganzes: gute Anfangs- und Schlußfigur in Abb. b. Vgl. S. 19 und S. 20.) $^1/_4$ n. Gr.

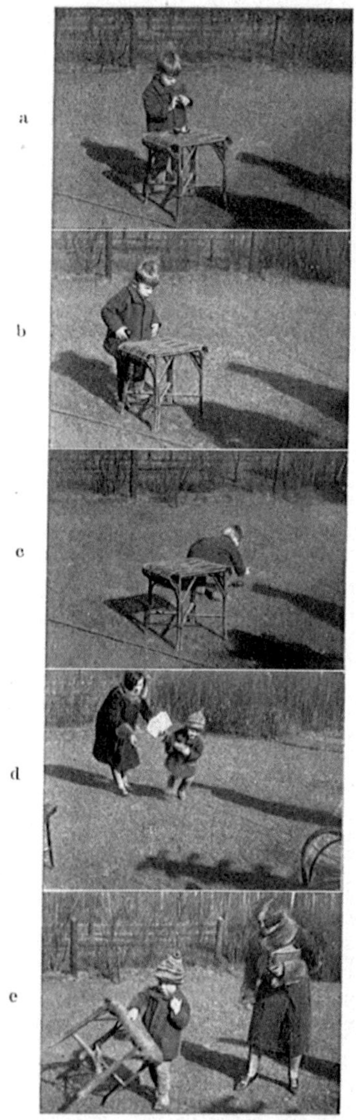

Abb. 6. Psychische Sättigung bei einem Dreijährigen. (Vgl. Text S. 18.)

Plate from Kurt Lewin, *The development of experimental psychology of the will and psychotherapy*, 1929.

Observing such repetitive actions as the tracing of a pentagram or a game played with building blocks, Lewin became interested in the phenomenon of 'psychic saturation' (*psychische Sättigung*).[4] The moment in which psychic saturation occurs is crucial to gestalt theory oriented by shape construction. It is the instant when the repetition of the same action or gesture suddenly faces a conflict: a 'psychic saturation' resulting in an excess or denial of action. Lewin speaks of '*Gestaltzerfall*'[5]—in German, the word *Zerfall* means decomposition, disintegration, or collapse—a decomposition of the shape occurring within the repetition of the gesture. This happens not as a consequence of the child's exhaustion, Lewin underlines, but results from an exhaustion of the field in which the gesture operates. He gives an example of the repetitive recitation of a poem which first unfolds a prolific variation of meaning, but soon leads to a decomposition of the entire poem into single words, '*forgetting, misspeaking, stutter*.'[6] Analysing different situations of such decompositions of *Gestalt*, Lewin points to the insufficiency of a model which opposes 'causality' and 'finality', 'drive' and 'will', as pure tendencies outlined differently in the works of Alfred Adler, Sigmund Freud, or Ludwig Klages. Instead, he posits a complex entanglement of 'field forces' and 'psychic tension systems' (*seelische Spannungssysteme*).[7]

But more crucially for the present context, Lewin derives his observations of *Gestalt* and *Gestaltzerfall* from an acute attention to the field: a milieu of action carefully framed in his experiments, mediated through the camera lens or circumscribed by the surface of the page itself in the case of tracings. Gestalt psychologists point to the importance of this milieu not only for the mediation of the action, but also and above all for its development, conceptualising it as a 'field' in which the forces can unfold. In this case, the mediation isolates and frames the field in which the action takes place.

Milieu and the Frame

In a similar way, one may be surprised to learn of the crucial role the frame played in Janmari's tracings. Janmari was an autistic, mute child entrusted to Deligny in 1967 at the age of twelve. He lived in the care network that Deligny created in Monoblet, in the Cévennes region, for twenty-five years.[8] As a child, he became one of the major figures in Deligny's theory and films. *Journal de Janmari (Janmari's Diary)* displays the tracings he produced between 2001 and 2002 during his weekly meetings with Gisèle Durand, who accompanied the children from the moment the network was created. The notebook reveals two different ways in which Janmari displayed shapes—small circles or waves—on the surface of a page. First, there are pages covered in shapes up to the margins; and second, there are those pages which contain a large figure—an ellipse or a rectangle—serving as a new frame for these circles or waves, and containing them. Gisèle Durand describes how she gave Janmari the first line for the frame, which was later replaced by a mere gesture completed by Janmari:

> Whenever I traced a vertical line from top to bottom, Janmari completed the rectangle by tracing the other three sides on his own. Soon I no longer needed to draw the line on the page. I just made the gesture in the air, and he drew all four sides. Then he set the pen down; I handed it back to him again, and he filled the frame with little circles and wavelets.[9]

The frame given by the surface of the page, which served as a milieu for Janmari's tracings, is replaced by an artificially constructed frame in which the repetition of the waves and circles can take place. It is not only the traced line, but also Durand's gesture, that are active elements in milieu construction and mediation.

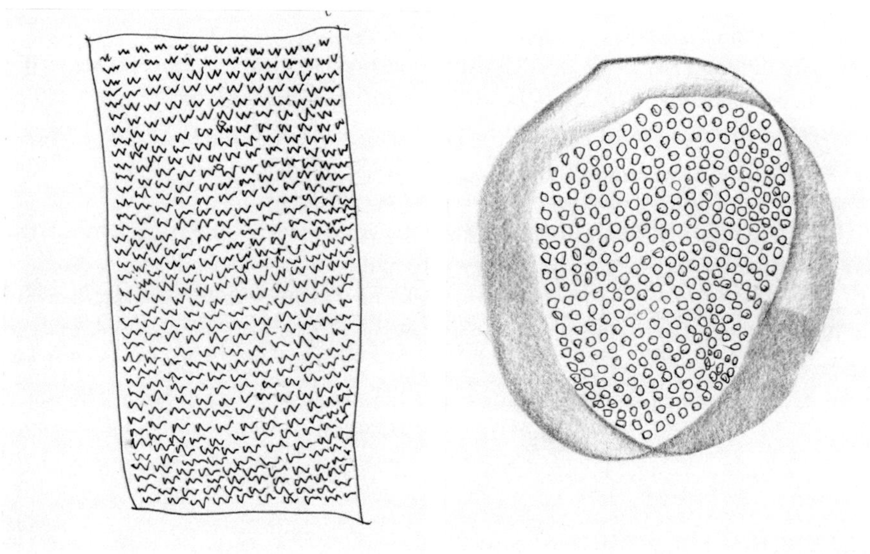

Lines traced on paper by Janmari, *Journal de Janmari,* L'Arachnéen, 2013. I thank in particular Sandra Alvarez de Toledo for generously providing these images.

Ce Gamin, là (*That Kid, There*), a film made by Renaud Victor and Deligny in 1975, shows a close-up of Janmari's small circles traced repeatedly, one beside the other, on a large sheet of paper. These tracings are followed by maps produced by the close presences which record Janmari's paths in a single day: 'He turns. He turns either around himself, the hands behind the back, one holding the other, or running.'[10] Deligny's voice-over makes the transition from the elliptic figures on paper to Janmari's repetitive circular movements in the meadows of the Cévennes. Thus the film montage produces a relation between these different milieus: Janmari's circles on paper, his trajectories in the space and his gestures. What the film's title suggests in the deictic, almost gestural mode of '*là*' reveals itself as a gesture of situating, an inscription of the milieu so important for Janmari.[11] Moreover, the film itself establishes a common ground through montage, creating a visual and dynamic field, a milieu, in which these different circles, these detours Janmari takes, coexist in their significant interrelation.

Janmari's tracings allude to one possible way in which mediation becomes part of milieu construction, a milieu in which the endless detours of an autistic gesture can emerge and unfold. For Deligny, this mediation process was intimately linked to a theoretical reflection on such autistic milieus and the practical camerawork in the Cévennes. One could even say that for him, media and milieus emerged simultaneously, enabling the actions and their detours. Thus media and milieus are closely related in their processual becoming, since mediation is a particular way of constructing the gaze. In this way, camering can be seen as a means of entering the logic of the milieu, becoming part of it while simultaneously maintaining a distance and taking its images. Marlon Miguel insightfully points to the relation between camering and '"gathering" (*recueillir*) or "catching" (*attraper*) images',[12] a process which resists the intentionality of filming in its traditional sense. This is how in 'Fossils Have a Hard Life: Apropos of the Image' Deligny abandons the notions of director or filmmaker in favour of the more impersonal and humble designation of 'image taker'. It is not a coincidence that the verb *camérer*, 'camering', resonates with *regarder*, 'looking', while replacing the authority of the subject with the accidental character of the milieu and its own temporality, envisioned by Deligny as camering 'the path of an iceberg and its thaw', as 'permanent cinema'.[13] Camering thus becomes an intransitive act involving the gaze into the process of uncovering a milieu.

Milieus of Minor Media

This becomes palpable in Deligny's work with the camera and his theory of the 'minor gesture'. *Le moindre geste* is one of the key concepts in Deligny's oeuvre. It serves as the title for a film produced collectively with Josée Manenti and Jean-Pierre Daniel, in collaboration with Aimé Agnel, Jean-Pierre Ruh, and Chris Marker, between 1962 and 1971 (*The Slightest Gesture*). It is also used in the title of a book: *Les Détours de l'agir ou le Moindre geste* (*The Detours of Acting or the Minor Gesture*). The work is multidimensional—at once a complex theoretical essay, an empirical observation, and a political stance towards the present. Deligny refers to a scene projected on screen that shows autistic children in their milieu of action. As if he were recovering the *optical unconscious* revealed by means of the camera, Deligny is far from reading these images as an immediate reflection of reality. For him, they instead bear traces of an irreducible singularity: '*le reste*' considered as 'residue' (*un résidu*), and more fundamentally as 'survival' (*une survivance*).[14] But 'survival' of what, one could ask.

Deligny answers this question dialectically: in this survival, relic, or 'atrophy', as he further describes the moment, he sees a fragment of a possible future, an outline or sketch ('*l'ébauche*') of what could be 'human'.[15]

Let us draw upon the way Deligny constructs his gaze, the way he opens his own observations directed towards an interaction between two autistic children, two girls, Isabelle and Anne.

> I don't disregard the tableau effect [*l'effet du tableau*] of this video screen on which I see the puddle, the stones, the two girls and their gestures, and farther, in a close-up, Anne's hands and Isabelle's hands, the same hands, whereas the gestures aren't the same at all.[16]

The scene described by Deligny becomes a seminal point in his text—a situation from which further elements derive and unfold.

> On seeing Isabelle and Anne crouched down, facing each other, a puddle, or rather, a hollow full of water, between them, one might think both are playing, so to speak. Anne grasps the stones along the edge of the crater one by one; she rinses them in the water. Her gesture seems to wash each stone until there is no earth on it, and each stone washed is put on the other side of the puddle. Isabelle observes attentively.
>
> Neither of them uses language. Isabelle hears, often understands, what is said. Anne is deaf to the meaning of words.[17]

Deligny's attentive gaze uncovers in Isabelle's gestures a form of play, while Anne's actions are of a different nature. While Isabelle inhabits different roles, helping or disturbing Anne's actions, Anne's gestures 'stumble on this obstacle, attempting to take up their own line again', what Deligny refers to as '*une ligne qui est ligne d'erre*'—'a line which is a wander line, a drift deriving from that *élan* where the other doesn't exist as other. [...] Anne doesn't play.'[18] To discover the difference between the two girls' gestures, it is necessary to trace the line of demarcation within their apparent interaction. Deligny looks again and again; the scene reappears several times in his text, each time generating new insights.

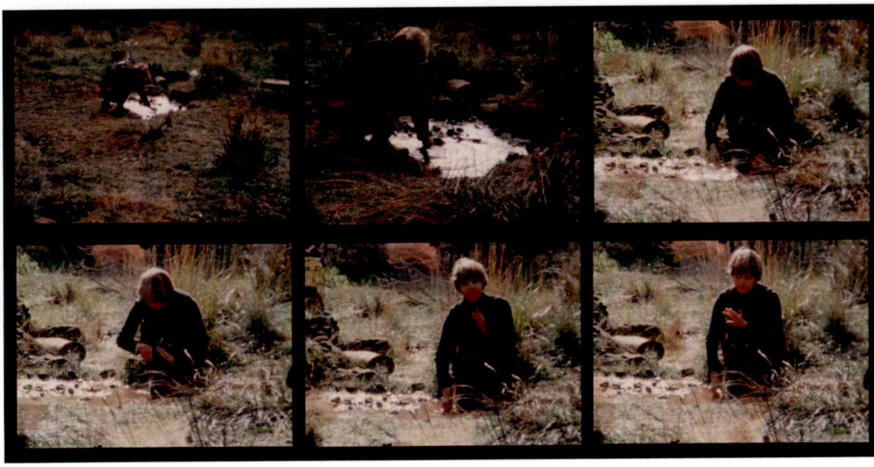

Anne in frames from super 8 rushes shot in the 1980s by Jacques Lin and Rose-Marie Ursenbacher. I would like to thank Martin Molina Gola and Marina Vidal-Naquet, who presented this material at ICI Berlin, for generously providing me with these images.

The camera—crucially conceptualised by Deligny as a 'pedagogical tool'[19] and thoroughly utilised in the Cévennes—virtually returns here, modelling Deligny's perspective on the scene, becoming part of his argument. In his text, it continues to serve as an analytical tool, providing a magnifying glass, a mediator of what Walter Benjamin once called 'heightened vividness' (*erhöhte Anschaulichkeit*).[20] The camera allowed Deligny to grasp what otherwise remains imperceptible to the capacity of vision, and in so doing 'to discover in the analysis of the individual moment the crystal of the total event'.[21] Repeatedly zooming in on the scene, Deligny's text recovers a plurality of milieus within the same frame, the same scene, which coexist, one beside the other. 'Isabelle is very close to Anne', he writes. Theirs are the same gestures, but while Isabelle is able to sneak into different roles, Anne avoids the obstacles introduced by Isabelle; her 'automated but subtle gestures' make it difficult to say 'her gestures' (*ses gestes*), as Deligny puts it, in favour of an impersonal and intransitive mode: Anne's gestures are *those gestures* (*ces gestes*).[22]

In *The Slightest Gesture*, several of these *minor gestures* appear. Indeed, they seem to be some sort of rite, as is the case, for example, with Yves's constant struggle to tie a knot. A gesture can be understood as a fundamentally intransitive act, an *infinitive*—that is, *to act* without finality or goal. What is the temporality of such acting which necessarily revolves in endless detours? How to locate or inscribe its movement within the materially defined conditions? For Deligny, this question goes hand in hand with a genuine refusal of a *primal* or *authentic* gesture. Both image and gesture are a matter of construction, inasmuch as they participate in the act of their mediation, which becomes an infinite process, *agir* rather than *faire*.[23] Such is the premise for Deligny's associating the intransitive gestures of autistic children with filming gestures, conceptualised via the French neologism *camérer*. Symptomatically, 'Mécréer', a text given the title of another such neologism—translated as 'Miscreating'—critically derives its origin from the verb *créer*, 'to create'.[24] In it, Deligny analyses the parallels between autistic gestures and filming gestures, revealing a crucial incommensurability which also traverses *The Slightest Gesture* as a leitmotiv. One of the film's central scenes can be read as a figuration for Deligny's understanding of autism and the use of film as an epistemic tool. He points out two events that happen simultaneously: two hands trying to knot a rope and a boy failing to climb out of a hole. Both scenes come to no end. While the tying of a knot stands for dramatic resolution, escaping from the hole delivers the matrix for a universal happy ending. But nothing happens. Instead, both actions idle in an infinite number of attempts. Deligny insists on the deceptive effect of such a scene, referring to his film's screening at the Cannes festival.

> Here one sees the difference between *camering* and making a film. The latter would be a question of providing the means with which to illuminate the pit so that one could follow the story and see the characters.
>
> Whereas with *camering*, the means are lacking, or nearly so. [...]
>
> To show two hands that aren't able to tie a knot is, without fail, to disappoint. That is why one must first deprive oneself, if only of the intention of being successful, of fulfilling the audience. Those two hands fiddling with the two ends of rope don't mean much.[25]

Deligny alludes here not only to the interrelation between medium and milieu but also to that between medium and action: *minor gestures* are entangled with and require some sort of *minor media* able to follow them and their 'detours of acting'. Hence, following the gestures of the two boys, the process of filming cannot help but participate in the logic of their movements. Deligny discovers here a double incommensurability: not only does the length of the scene exceed that of a classic drama, thereby deceiving the expectations of each potential viewer, but the boy's failing to tie a knot exceeds any economy of means, confronting Deligny with the sheer impossibility of filming the scene. At the same time, the excessive temporality of the action points to a stunning coexistence of *different milieus* within one frame, one field of vision. In the autistic person's 'wander line' or 'minor gesture', Deligny sees the necessity of filming, of making *those gestures* visible in their singularity. Here Deligny operates similarly to Soviet filmmakers such as Sergei Eisenstein, Esfir Shub, or Dziga Vertov, who worked with non-professional actors, the so-called *tipazh*, to reveal the irreducible marks of a particular social class.

In both cases, filming goes hand in hand with a crucial de-dramatisation and 'de-anecdotisation' of the action, to quote one of the key concepts Eisenstein used in the 1920s to allude to this new mode of filmmaking. This cinema had to learn from the 'physiological quality of the detail', rather than from the shiny figure of the main actor. In this sense, Eisenstein argued for a general 'de-anecdotisation' of a particular case—a hero or a star—in favour of the intensity of a 'close-up', and 'the expression of the theme through a strong impact of the material'.[26] He argued for revealing the micro-drama of a gesture instead of the macro-drama of a happy ending, the singularity of a facial expression rather than the glamour of a character. This is a further meaning of *minor*, which comes close to Deligny's network in the Cévennes: a milieu where other—as yet non-visible—milieus can emerge.

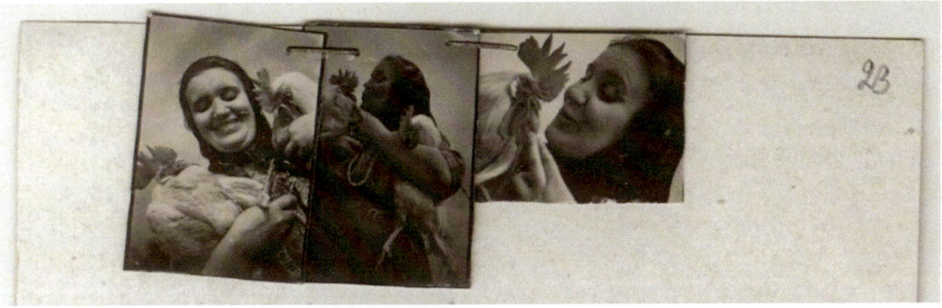

Casting cards portraying non-professional actors (*tipazh*) for Sergei Eisenstein's film *Bezhin Meadow* (1935–37), Russian State Archive for Literature and Art, Moscow.

In contrast to playing a role, such *acting* in and through film involves the milieu in a double sense: firstly, as a materially and historically produced *lieu*, a place with its particular structure, architecture, and temporality; and secondly, milieu as an extension of the intransitive action: as potentiality, a *lieu* of manifold coexisting *milieux* where Deligny sees a medium for new forms of collectivity. This understanding of cinema coincides with Eisenstein's claim for a cinema 'beyond the stars', a cinema operating with non-professional actors. Eisenstein's short text 'Beyond the Stars', which ascribes its own meaning to the term *tipazh*, can be associated with Deligny's *minor gesture*.[27] Eisenstein's ironically promotional text recommends releasing *Battleship Potemkin* in America, describing it as a 'film without stars'. 'The absence of "stars" as Eisenstein writes, was a reason why attention within this work turned to countless cinematographic problems that ordinarily, under the conditions of the protagonists' "starlight" in other productions, invariably remain in the shadows.'[28] That these 'cinematographic problems' need to be considered in terms of their political consequences—as problems of aesthetic figuration of a radical singularity—can likewise be understood as a central issue of Deligny's work.

The endless detours of the labyrinth addressed in the beginning appear in this context not as the negative figure of an infinity to be overcome, but rather as a potentiality, a dialectical chance to recover the difference within the repetition. Detours of acting become synonymous with a mode of existence within a milieu and its simultaneous unity and multiplicity—a milieu of endless milieus.

Notes

1 Fernand Deligny, *The Arachnean and Other Texts*, translated by Drew S. Burk and Catherine Porter, Minneapolis, Univocal Publishing, 2015, p. 62, translation slightly modified. In French Deligny makes use of two terms to allude to two different modalities of being: l'humain (the human) positively embraces the human in all its differences and singularities, including autism, while l'homme-qui-nous-sommes (the Man-that-we-are) refers rather critically to the humanist individual distinguished by rationality and carried by the teleology of progress.

2 Intertitles from Kurt Lewin's film *Field Forces as Impediments for a Performance*, 1929.

3 Kurt Lewin, *Die Entwicklung der experimentellen Willenspsychologie und die Psychotherapie*, Leipzig, S. Hirzel, 1929. Lewin first presented this research at the Third Medical Congress of Psychotherapy in 1929.

4 *Ibid.*, p. 14; figures 1 to 5.

5 *Ibid.*, p. 17; figures 1 to 5. Lewin derives the term *Gestaltzerfall* from a study on linguistic recitation phenomena analysed in H. P. Weld and V. J. Don, 'Lapse of Meaning with Visual Fixation', *American Journal,* vol. 35, No. 3, p. 446, 1924.

6 *Ibid.*, p. 17.

7 *Ibid.*, p. 22.

8 See Gisèle Durand, Postface to *Journal de Janmari*, Paris, L'Arachnéen, 2013.

9 *Ibid.*

10 Fernand Deligny, Renaud Victor, *Ce Gamin, là*, 1975.

11 In 'Mécréer' Deligny speaks of the adverb 'là' as referring to 'milieux et lieux repérables', a concrete locus of the network in Monoblet with its specific landscape and architecture.

12 Marlon Miguel, Introduction, *supra*, p. 37. See also Deligny's text 'Fossils Have a Hard Life: Apropos of the Image,' *supra*, p. 155.

13 Fernand Deligny, 'Camering' [1978–1983], *supra*, p. 167.

14 Fernand Deligny, 'Les Détours de l'agir ou le Moindre geste', in Fernand Deligny, *Œuvres*, Paris, L'Arachnéen, 2007, p. 1249.

15 Idem.

16 *Ibid.*, p. 1252.

17 *Ibid.*, p. 1251.

18 *Ibid.*, p. 1251.

19 Fernand Deligny, 'The Camera, a Pedagogical Tool', *supra*, pp. 57-61.

20 Walter Benjamin, *The Arcades Project*, ed. Rolf Tiedemann, New York, Belknap Press, 2002, p. 641.

21 Idem.

22 Fernand Deligny, 'Les Détours de l'agir ou le Moindre geste', in Œuvres, op. cit., p. 1252.

23 Idem.

24 See *supra*, p. 78, p. 86.

25 Fernand Deligny, 'Miscreating', supra, p. 80.

26 This article consists of Eisenstein's answers to a questionnaire, published in a newspaper and later reprinted under the title 'Literatura i kino' [Literature and Cinema], in Izbrannye proizvedenia, vol. 5, 6 vols., Moscow, Isskustvo, 1968, pp. 525–529. See also Elena Vogman, *Dance of Values. Sergei Eisenstein's Capital Project*, Zurich, Diaphanes, 2019.

27 Sergei Eisenstein, *Metod*, ed. Naum Kleiman, vol. 1, Moscow, Muzei Kino, 2002, p. 33.

28 *Ibid.*

Kolibri 360 GmbH
Ferdinand-Jühlke-Straße 7
99095 Erfurt, Deutschland
produktsicherheit@kolibri360.de